Eyebrow Shaping And Colouring To Suit Face Shapes

Edition 7

By Robyna Smith-Keys

ISBN-13: 978-0-9945693-3-2
Black and White Copy

Published By Robyna Smith-Keys

May 2014

Revised September 2015
Edition 6 Revised February 2016
Edition 7 Revised July 2016
By Robyna at Beauty School Books
http://www.beautyschoolbooks.com
Email beautyschoolbooks.com
Follows Industry Standards
SHBBFAS001 - Provide lash and brow services

Copyright

at Beauty School Books

Published by Robyna Smith-Keys

If you have purchased the EBook Copy -

You may load it onto two computers owned by you. Your computer IP Address with be returned to me.

PREAMBLE

When I began writing this book, my intention was for Hairdressing and Beauty salon operators to be able to improve on their skills at eye enhancement treatments to suit face shapes. However, as time goes by and with each book revision, I have also tried to make the information a suitable read for everyone.

Eyebrows shape our face and enhance our natural appearance. No matter how much or how little eye makeup we wear, if our eyebrows have no shape or colour our face as we age can look tired and older.

Due to the fact, that this book is more suited to a student than a home user, there are things far and beyond shape and colour that you need to understand. Yet, I have tried mainly to set you in the right direction of exploring eyebrow shapes and colour to suit face shapes, skin tones and undertones. I have sought to do without making this book too long and wordy.

Knowing what to do for each client, as time goes by, your passion for becoming great will become second nature. Getting through that journey hopefully will become shorter by the thought provoking information contained herein this book. You cannot expect to become a great eye enhancement technician with little to no training.

You cannot expect this book to land in your lap with all the knowledge and mind tools you will need to become an expert. You can, however, expect after reading this book to be set on the right journey to understanding eyebrow shaping to suit face shapes.

It will depend largely on how much time you are prepared to spend researching the face shapes of people and their eyebrow shape, their hair type and skin tones and undertones.

After fifty years in the industry, I myself, am passionately, still learning.

Always be guided by a clients wants and needs. After the initial learning process, you will feel you know it all and can forget:-

It is not about you. It is about the client.
It is about what they are comfortable with.
It is about how they see themselves in the mirror.

Note: Point of view will switch from the first person to the third person throughout this book. Grammar and punctuation will not be of the finest, and I make no apologies for that.

While ever I am alive and still of sound mind I am happy to answer a question or two via email. It must be about the topic of the book that you have purchased from my website. I have found questions point out the weak areas in my books. Your questions and comments assist me to improve on the next addition. That, in turn, helps others.

TABLE OF CONTENTS

Eyebrow Shaping & Colouring To Suit Face Shapes

BEFORE WE BEGIN

Before we begin to consider a new shape or colour for a clients eyebrows, we must explore their likes and dislikes. Fill in all the Client Forms and take their before photo.

If you are a home user trying to improve your look, all this information can be daunting. The simple answer is you have a curved brow bone that your eyebrows are positions on. Providing your brow bone is not damaged, follow the upper side of the contour of your brow bone. That is how I teach people that are blind to apply powered eyebrow shadow. Most of us have a slight indent in that bone where the contour should peak. As does our check bone and that is where rouge/ blush should start.

May I suggest.

Gather photos of yourself.

Pick out two photos of yourself where you looked your loveliest.

What colour was your hair?

What style was your hair?

What colour were your eyebrows?

Were your eyebrows an attractive shape in those two photos?

Make a copy of those photos, get some paint and try a few different eyebrow shapes and colours with kids paint. On each photo have one eyebrow shaped one way and the other eyebrow shaped a different way.

You could take these photos to your Hairdresser and your Beauty Therapist to help them recapture your beauty.

When we follow all the rules, sometimes we are not comfortable with the look. As we age, our face shape changes and adjustments to colour and shape need to change as well.

It is important to play with hair styles and eyebrow shapes and colour. This is the best way to develop your most youthful look.

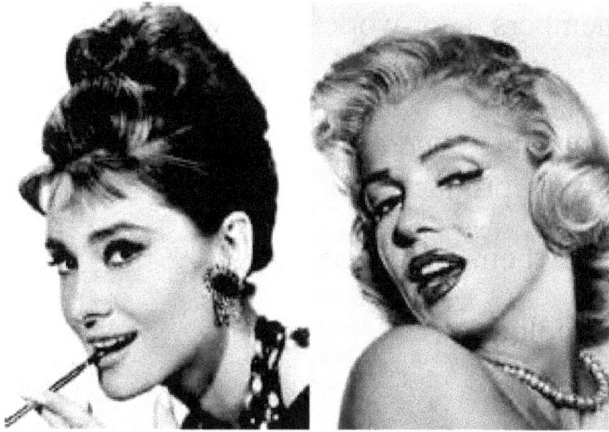

FIGURE 1 MARILYN & AUDREY

Have a look at Marilyn Monroe and Audrey Hepburn. They have similar eyebrows with totally different looks. In this next photo, Marilyn looks more sophisticated and lady-like due to her hairstyle.

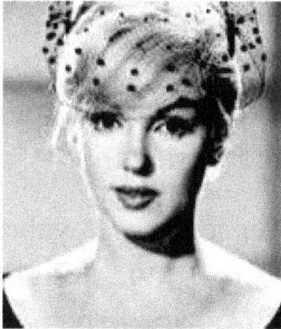

If you intend to develop a method of designing eyebrows to suit face shapes, you will need to practice and gain experience by gathering friends and family members and work your way through this book.

1. Know and understand all the available eyebrow products.

2. Check their face shape.

3. Hair colour.

4. Original hair colour

5. Skin tones and undertones.

6. Eyebrow shaping.

Use the diagram and the instruction in this book.

Gather friends and have a girly day and have some fun.

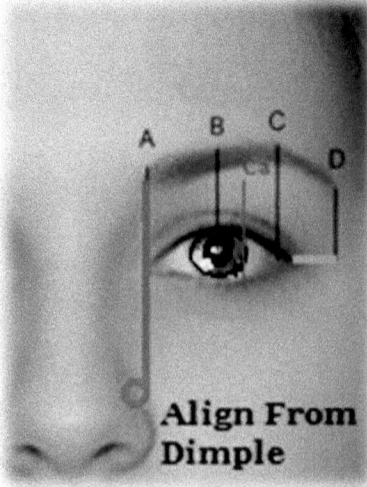

Take before and after (photo) shots.

You could use eyebrow powders to design a few shapes on each person before you begin shaping their eyebrows with wax or tweezers.

Align From Dimple

I like to buy a combination of powdered shadows for a soft eyebrow look. Using pencils and gels takes a lot of practice. Powder eyebrow shaper is quick and easy for a home user to use and should be sold in every salon. Who is best to demonstrate to a client how to use a powder shaper, than you her beauty therapist? I use Elizabeth Ardens Clinique have a

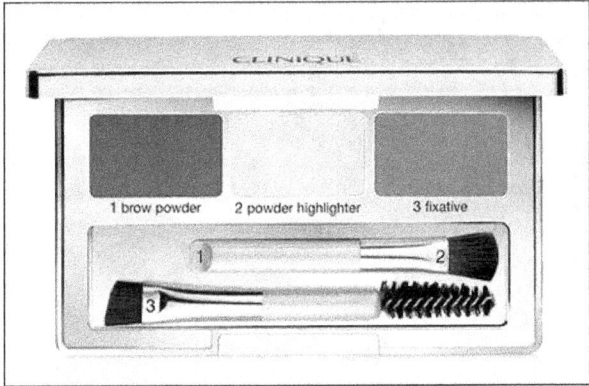

great one as well. I like this tutorial on Youtube:-

https://www.youtube.com/watch?v=D8A2-W17AME

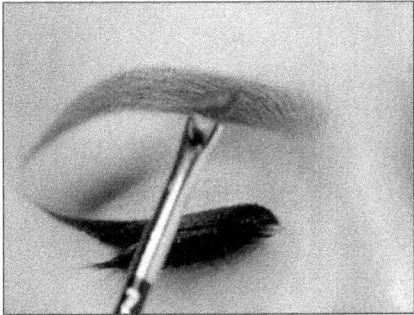

Personally. I think she would look better with a bit more definition near the nose bridge, to soften the nose ridge. Two shades of brown would also give a

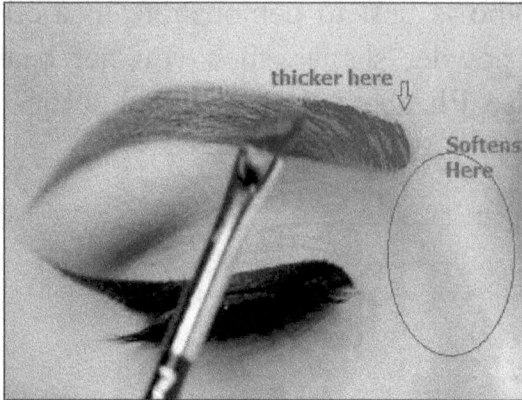

thicker here

Softens Here

more natural look

EYEBROWS

Eyebrows are one of the most important features of a person's face. When your eyebrows are the wrong shape for your face, you will look tired or older than you should.

On the other hand, eyebrows that are the right colour and shape, to suit your face shape and hair colour will enhance your beauty. Thus, giving your face, a dimension without makeup.

Experts can tell just by looking at your eyebrows

whether they are the right shape for your face or not. How do you tell if a client or your own eyebrows have the wrong shape:-

- You don't have an arch to your brow.

- Your eyebrows end too soon.

- Your eyebrows don't grow close to the bridge of your nose.

- They grow over the bridge of your nose.

- You can never figure out where your eyebrows should start and where they should end.

- You have pale eyebrows

- You have different shape eyebrows.

- People often ask if you are tired

- People seldom say you look great.

If you've experienced any of these issues, you probably don't have the right eyebrow shape or colour for your type of face.

At this point and before we begin the study of face and eyebrow shapes I feel it is important to take a little about the human body and the symmetrical issues we all face and why.

SYMMETRICAL ISSUES

Before we begin the art of shaping and colouring eyebrows and eyelashes to suit face shapes, there are a few things to consider.

First, our bodies are not symmetrical.

Second, everyone has different skin types, skin tones, undertones and pigment structures.

Third, we are human. Therefore, everyone is controlled by different circumstances and sufferings. Governed by where, when and to whom we were born. The human mind is very delicate and extremely complex.

What you think looks good on a client may not be what she or he is comfortable with.

MASCULINE AND FEMININE SIDES OF THE BODY

If you look in the mirror and view your profile from each side, you may notice that the two sides of your face are slightly different from one another.

Each eyebrow will be slightly different.

I thought you might like to read this article.

Additionally, your left hand is similar to but different from your right hand. In fact, these subtle differences pervade both sides of your entire body. Considering these differences in the context of the idea that the right side of your body is masculine and the left side feminine may shed some light on how balanced you are in relation to your masculine and feminine qualities.

Intuition, feelings, openness, and unselfishness govern the feminine side of our natures. The masculine side is characterised by logic, facts, systems, and self-interest. If you are giving too much to others to the detriment of yourself, your feminine side may be overactive, and your right side may need strengthening, to speak up on your behalf, protecting and conserving your energy. If your life is too rigidly structured, your masculine aspect may be overactive; developing your feminine aspect will bring a more open-ended and creative approach.

One day in 1788, students at the Hunterian School of Medicine in London were opening a cadaver when they discovered something startling. The dead man's anatomy was a mirror image of normal. His liver was on his left side instead of the right. His heart had beaten on his right side, not his left.

The students had never seen anything like it, and they rushed to find their teacher, the Scottish physician Matthew Baillie, who was just as stunned as they were. "It is so extraordinary as scarcely to have been seen by any of the most celebrated anatomists," he later wrote.

His report was the first detailed description of the condition, which came to be known as situs inversus and is thought to occur in about 1 in 20,000 people. Baillie argued that if doctors could figure out how this strange condition came to be, they might come to understand how our bodies normally tell the right side from the left.

Over two centuries later, the mystery of left and right still captivates scientists.

"I know what it is, you know what it is, but how does the embryo learn what it is?" asked Dominic P. Norris, a developmental biologist at the Medical Research Council in Harwell, England.

Now Dr. Norris and other scientists are beginning to answer that question. They have pinpointed some of the steps by which embryos' organs develop on the left or right. Their research may do more than simply solve an old puzzle.

Mutations that cause situs inversus can lead to a number of serious disorders, including congenital heart defects. Deciphering the effects of mutated genes could lead to diagnoses and treatments for those conditions.

"Understanding how you put this axis together has a lot of implications for understanding congenital heart disease," said Rebecca Burdine, a molecular biologist at Princeton.

Our bodies start out symmetrical, the left side a perfect reflection of the right. "Visible signs of left-right asymmetry in the human body are apparent around six weeks," said Sudipto Roy of the Institute of Molecular and Cell Biology in Singapore, an author of a review of left-right asymmetry that was published last week in the journal Open Biology.

The heart shows the first visible asymmetry. Starting out as a simple tube, it loops to the left. The heart then starts to grow different structures on each side, producing the chambers and vessels required to pump blood.

Meanwhile, other organs start moving. The stomach and liver each move clockwise away from the midline of the embryo. The large intestines sprout an appendix on the right. The right lung grows three lobes, the left only two.

Nevertheless, these visible changes arise long after the embryo has developed differences on its left and right. Experiments have revealed that the early embryo produces different proteins on each side while it still looks symmetrical.

Biologists have pinpointed a single spot where this symmetry breaking starts: a tiny pit called the node, on the embryo's midline. The interior of the node is lined with hundreds of tiny hairs, called cilia, which whirl round and round at a rate of 10 times a second.

These whirling cilia are tilted, pointing away from the head. The tilt is essential to their ability to divide the body into left and right. Recently Kathryn V. Anderson and her colleagues at Memorial Sloan-Kettering Cancer Center disabled genes required to tip the cilia in the node. As they report in the journal Development, that mutation led to some mouse embryos' developing a mirror-image anatomy.

The tilt of the cilia is so important because the embryo is bathed, in a thin film of fluid; if they were upright, they would push the fluid in all directions, creating no flow at all. "It's like a blender," Dr Norris said. "It just goes round and round." Tilted, they all push the fluid in one direction, from right to left. When scientists reversed that flow in mouse embryos, it resulted in reversed organs.

It takes only a very weak flow to the left side to start an embryo on its proper development: Last year, scientists at Osaka University in Japan reported that the whirling of just two cilia were enough to get the job done.

And that raises another question: "What on earth are we doing with all those cilia if we don't need them?" as Dr Norris put it. "We don't know."

Once the fluid starts flowing, it takes only three or four hours for the left and right sides to be determined. Scientists have only a patchy understanding of the steps in between.

In the first step, the fluid flows across the node until it reaches the left side of the rim. The rim is ringed by cilia that do not spin. Somehow, they respond to the flow. They may physically bend, or the flow may deliver some protein to them. "We don't know the nitty-gritty," Dr. Norris said. "We don't know the actual mechanics in these cells of what is happening."

Regardless of those details, the cilia on the rim of the node respond to the flow — possibly by releasing calcium atoms that then spread to surrounding cells. Those cells respond by spewing out a protein called Nodal, which spreads through the left side of the embryo, in turn spurring other cells to spew out Nodal of their own in a kind of feedback loop that leaves the left side loaded with Nodal and the right with almost none. "Nodal begets Nodal, and then we're off," Dr. Norris said.

Scientists are still working out how Nodal helps determine the anatomy on each side of the body. In recent years, many researchers have focused not on mice but on zebra fish, which have the advantage of having transparent embryos; cells in the embryos can be engineered to glow so the organs can be observed taking shape.

Dr. Burdine, at Princeton, studies how Nodal shapes the anatomy of the zebrafish heart as embryonic cells migrate around the organ. "Nodal seems to be directly telling the cells on the left side to move faster than the ones on the right," she said.

As she and her colleagues reported in the January issue of PLoS Genetics, the fast-moving cells on the left side drag the entire heart clockwise. From that initial twist, the heart then develops its distinctive left and right sides.

Some studies suggest that these early signals also influence brain development. Scientists have long known that the two sides of the human brain have some important differences. The right hemisphere, for example, plays a big role in understanding the mental lives of other people; the left hemisphere is important for focusing attention. Other vertebrates also have left-right brain differences, but the origins of the imbalance are mostly a mystery.

"I think that in vertebrates, it is zebra fish where we know the most details," said Joshua T. Gamse, a biologist at Vanderbilt University. Dr. Gamse and other researchers have found that Nodal prompts a small part of the fish's brain to grow differently on the left and right sides. That difference then radiates outward to other parts of the brain. But it is not clear whether humans and other mammals develop in a similar fashion. As they look at these biological signals, scientists are also studying disorders that may be tied to their disruption.

Situs inversus, the complete flip of the organs that Baillie described in 1788, may be the most dramatic of these disorders, but it is also one of the most harmless.

"People can walk around with their axis completely inverted, and no one knows until your doctor figures out your heart's not where it should be," Dr. Burdine said.

The reversal is relatively safe because all the organs line up with one another. "You look at yourself in the mirror, and you look perfectly normal," Dr. Norris said. "You don't stop looking like a human being just because you see yourself backwards."

The real danger, it appears, is in incomplete reversals — "when you get a confusion, when you get things not quite meeting," as Dr. Norris put it.

Most worrisome are cases in which the heart is affected. "If you put the heart in the wrong place, and everything else is correct," Dr. Burdine said, "that's almost always fatal."

In other cases, the heart grows correctly on the left side of the body, but the structures inside the heart — the valves and chambers — grow on the wrong side. These disorders may not be immediately fatal, but they can become dangerous later in life, requiring complex surgery to rearrange the heart.

Dr. Burdine hopes that research on left-right disorders will lead to genetic tests that can predict the risk of these hidden heart defects. She even sees an

application to attempts to rebuild damaged hearts
with stem cells.

"It's going to be more than just making the right
cells," she said, adding that they would need to be
placed in the proper three-dimensional structure and
given the correct signals on where to go.

"And one of those signals," she said, "is the left-right
signal."

This article has been revised to reflect the following
correction:

Correction: June 5, 2013

An article on Tuesday about asymmetry in the human
body misstated the scientific affiliation of Dominic
Norris, a developmental biologist who has studied
the steps by which embryos' organs develop on the
left or right. Dr. Norris is with the Medical Research
Council in Harwell, England, not Cambridge
University.

Credit:- http://www.nytimes.com/2013/06/04/science/growing-
left-growing-right-how-a-body-breaks-
symmetry.html?pagewanted=all&_r=0

NO ARCH TO YOUR BROW.

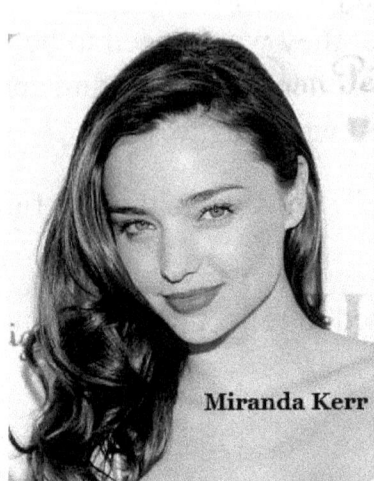

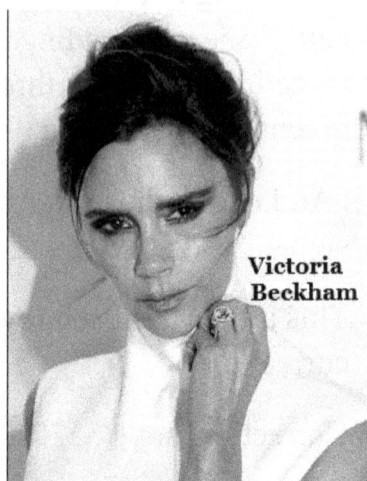

Victoria
Beckham

Miranda Kerr

Miranda Kerr looks fine with her no arch brows due to her youthful appearance. They do however, make her forehead look as though it is bulging out in a moon shape. A tapering, whippy fringe could rectify that situation. Her photographer should have encouraged her to lift her head a little for this shot. Her pretty yet cheeky face at this stage in her life allows this fault to go unnoticed by most people.

Victoria on the other hand definitely is at the age, where she needs to consider an arched or peaked brow. If for any other reason, other than health issues Victoria could do with a bit more beef to flatter her pretty face.

However in a salon situation, you would not mention these issues unless the client asked for your professional advice.

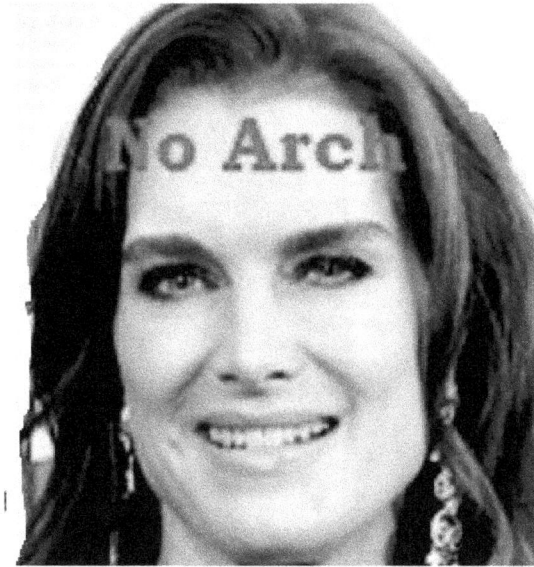

In the above photo, the eyebrows have no arch. They have a peak on the outer edge of the eye. The eyebrow tint / colour is a perfect match for her hair colour and skin tone. Her lipstick is way too light even for day wear.

I have drawn some lines on the next photo to show how her eyebrows could be improved.

I do not have a drawing program so the drawing is not great, but you should be able to gauge the difference.

If you look at both photos from a distance, you will get a better idea.

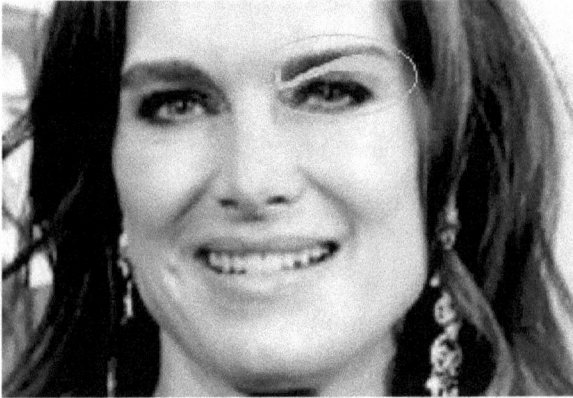

By removing some of the inner eyebrows and removing some of the brows from under the inner eye area, her eyes would appear less dropped. I was unable to draw it in, but I would also add a dash more height to her inner eyebrow upper section. This would add some gentle movement to her forehead.

Eyebrows are to be designed to create a more youthful look. Some clients may not like their new look straight away but when a few people say things like:

"What have you done ? You look younger."

Or " Did you change your hair colour?"

People are not always able to put their finger on what is different, but they do know that something has changed for the better. That is when your client will settle into her new look and enjoy it.

If you or your client does not have an arch to the eyebrow, then there are several ways to create one. Remember everyone is asymmetrical / lopsided. Both sides of your face are different.

A Beauty Therapist needs to study many face shapes and skin types and their learning is ongoing. With some types of eyebrows, it is possible to change the shape with careful waxing techniques. Pencil and brow powders can be used to create an arch. Also, a good Cosmetic tattooist can be appointed to tattoo a wonderful full shape or to add the look of a few hair like strokes to create the arch look.

A good beauty therapist is always ready to improve the look of her client thus improving the confidence of her client. If you are trying to change your own look, a beauty therapist or makeup artist should be engaged to assist you with good pencilling techniques. The pencil will come off during the day, or when you swim. However, you can always carry an eyebrow pencil with you and very quickly reapply. I myself prefer Elizabeth Arden's eyebrow powder sold in a compact with mirror.

WHEN OUR EYEBROWS END TOO SOON.

The answer here is similar to above. You can either use a pencil or engage a Cosmetic tattooist.

You can also have a hair implant. I am not in favour of the implant method as there is a tiny noticeable hair knot at the base of each hair. An Eyebrow infill can also have a knotty look. However, for people with bald patched an infill works wonders.

NO EYEBROWS CLOSE TO THE NOSE BRIDGE.

When eyebrows don't grow, close to the bridge of the nose.

The answer is the same engage a cosmetic tattooist or use a pencil to fill in the missing hairs. Have your Beauty Therapist or a makeup artist show you how or look into the mirror and practice using a pencil to fill the shape in. Remember practice makes perfect. It is small light feather-like strokes, and you must take your time in good light, and a magnifying mirror is best.

EYEBROWS SHOULD START AND END.

If you can never figure out where your eyebrows should start and where they should end . You probably don't have the right eyebrow shape for your face, and that is easily fixed with waxing and tinting.

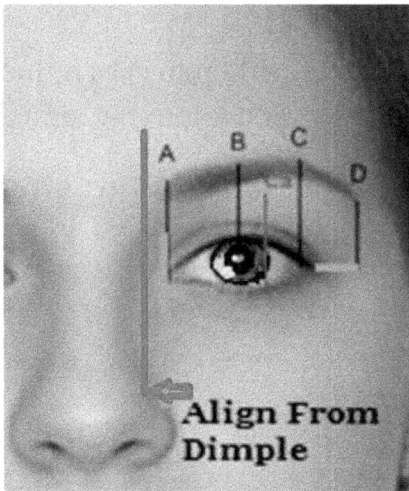

Align From Dimple

A.   Will always start in line with either the outer edge of the nose or if you have a wide nose, start the line from the dimple in your nose .

B.   The eyebrow should have slightly tapered as you reach the B mark, which is the centre of your eye pupil.

C. Position "C: is for a peaked type of arch. The peak should be almost at the end of the eyelid outer corner.

D. The end of the brow should be a thumb space away from the outer corner of the eyelid or half the width of your nose.

Ca. A curved arch should be lined up to start at the end of the pupil. Be sure the client is looking straight ahead.

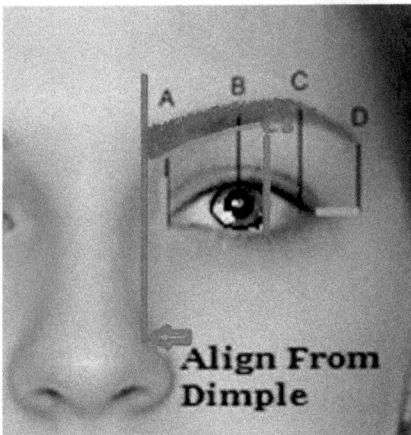

Align From
Dimple

Compare the two alignment photos. Everyone will have a different opinion. In this second photo I have filled in her brow from the dimple, alignment and the inner eye edge "A" plus I gave her a slightly thicker and darker brow. This I believe sends the focus away from her broad nose tip to the centre of the nose.

Am I right or am I wrong. This would be an option; you could give a client and have them decide. The first photo with the wider gap between eyebrows, is softer, but the focus is on her nose tip.

With my eyebrows on my right side I follow the nature hair growth. On my left side I add colour to the underside of my peak as my left brow tail sits higher than the tail on my right brow.

Remember there is no two faces that are identical shapes. Therefore the shaping rules are **not** set in concrete.

To assist a mature face- look younger, you do not always lift the brow, by removing hair from under the brow.

Sometimes you need to add a line with powder shader or cosmetic tattooing to the underside of the brow. I could give you a million photos of eyebrow shapes and ways to shape each or show you those million photos with three different ways to shape each person's eyebrows and there would still be more information you would require.

Eyebrow Shaping & Colouring To Suit Face Shapes

Learn the basics and use your sixth sense to glamorise a person's face. Practice on family and friends.

Offer your client an eyebrow tidy up or a full consultation for an eye enhancement treatment.

- Eyebrow Wax $21

- Eyebrow Tint $21

- Eyelash and Eyebrow Tint $32.50

- Eyebrow Wax And Tint $29.50

- Eyebrow Wax and Tint Plus Eyelash Tint $43.50

- Eyebrow Enhancement with Consultation $79
- Special On Tuesday $55.50
- Add a mini pedicure or manicure while you are here for just $26.50

Prices will be different in each Country, Town or City.

As well as your time and products, you need to factor into your price list; the cost of Rent, Insurance, equipment, cleaning, reception staff, water, electricity, telephone and advertising.

The above prices are what they charge 2016 on the Gold Coast in Australia. All things considered, overall, this is a low priced service you are offering. Therefore, you need to be well trained, fast and yet extremely good at eyebrow styling to gain repeat business. You should also develop the skills to sell products and more services to your client.

EYEBROW ENHANCEMENT WITH CONSULTATION

Now this is where you gain a clients trust forever.

Ask them to bring some photos of them self to the appointment. The photos should be at various stages in their life. Have a good look at how they have been grooming their eyebrows over the last 10-20 years.

Measure their face, eyebrows and discover their face shape.

Use pencils and eyebrow powders to create a few different shapes.

It is their life, their face and you need to be, guided by their feelings.

All this should take you no more than 25 minutes. Time is money.

LOW ARCH EYEBROWS

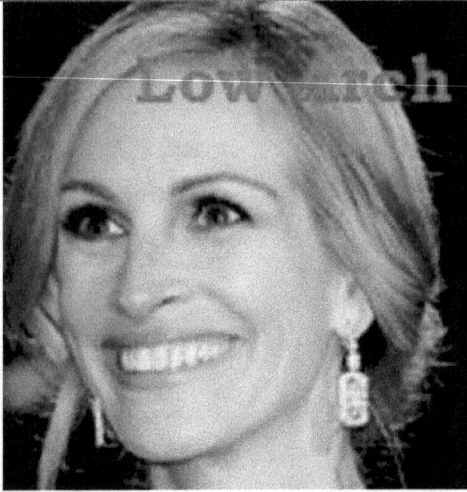

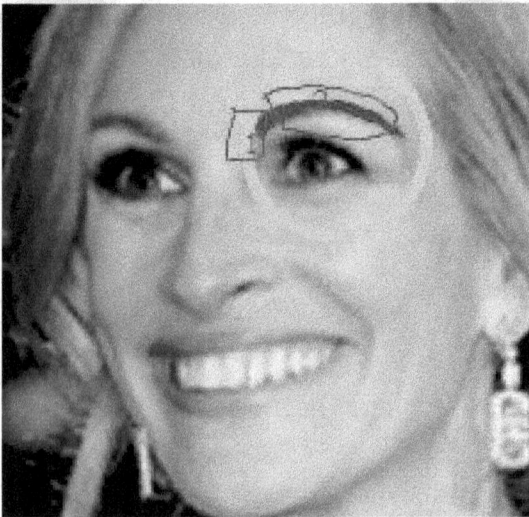

Because of the shape and size of Julia's mouth, she needs slightly thicker eyebrows. Which brings me to the point that if your client is going to have a lip filler, then she or he is best to first have an eyebrow tidy up. Then return after the lip filler treatment for an eyebrow enhancement treatment.

Your clients will be well advised, to have their eyebrow styling session after a new hair colour and definitely, after the lip filler has been applied.

1. She needs the inner part of the brow slightly removed. I did this in the program "Paint", which limits my demonstration abilities, but I feel you will get my idea.

2. Her upper height needs to be, added to.

3. Her eyebrow tint needs to be taupe for this hair colour.

4. Julia has a large space from the outer edge of her eyes to the outside tip of her eyebrow. Therefore, Julia should also wear a light brown or pinkish shadow in this area.

5. Her brow is too long, and the outer taper needs to be decreased. With the outer tip slightly lifted.

6. I also added colour to the underside of her brow

In this next photo of Julia I have tried with my limited drawing skill to demonstrate:-

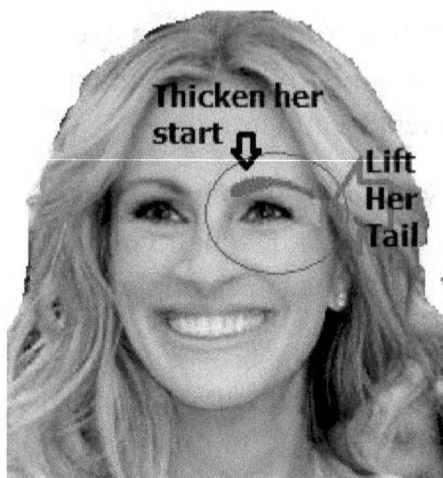

Julia's eyes look larger and brighter and her nose tip softer, with a thicker brow.

I added eyebrow colour closer to her nose , lifted her eyebrow tail and thickened her brow.

I wish I could spend a day with her. When she lightens her hair, she needs some dark chocolate foils around the front. Blonde hair is not her most flattering colour. This strawberry blonde is wrong for her complexion.

Mmm, I am not completely happy with that eyebrow shape, on Julia , but I am limited by the tools I have. However, my main point is you need to play with eyebrow powders and concealer before you decide what looks best for a client or yourself. The right eyebrow on the left side of this picture makes her face look flat. The right eyebrow gives her face a more plump healthy look and lifts her cheeks. Look at half the face at a time and you decide.

ARCH AND BROW TOO THIN

By adding more eyebrow closer to the nose and thickening the brow at the top the lines under her eyes are less noticeable. Plus she needs some ash-tint hue added to the eyebrow tint. Her eyebrows need feathering which I am unable to demonstrate with my drawing tools.

Photo Credit   Alberto E. Rodriguez

Check how the left eyebrow (right eyebrow as you view the photo}now gives her eye more depth and sparkle.

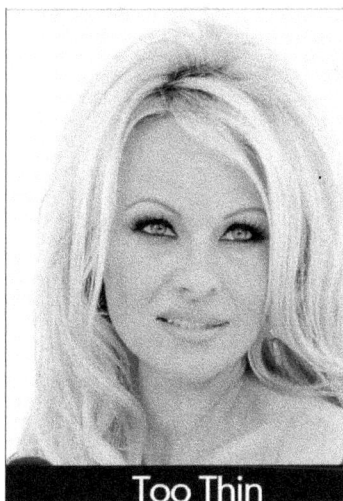

Too Thin

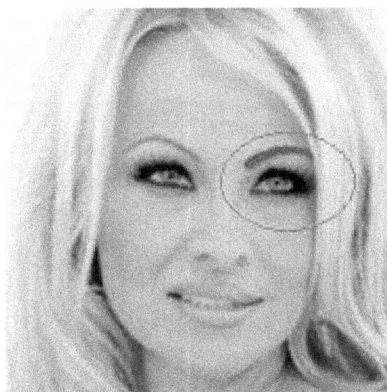

THICK EYEBROWS

MY FAVOURITE ACTRESS ELIZABETH TAYLOR

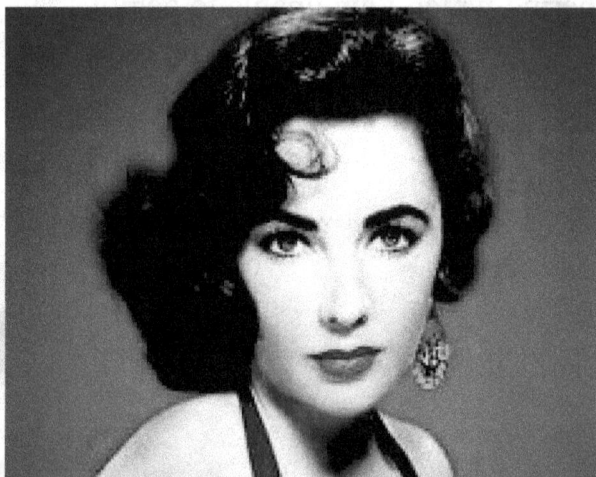

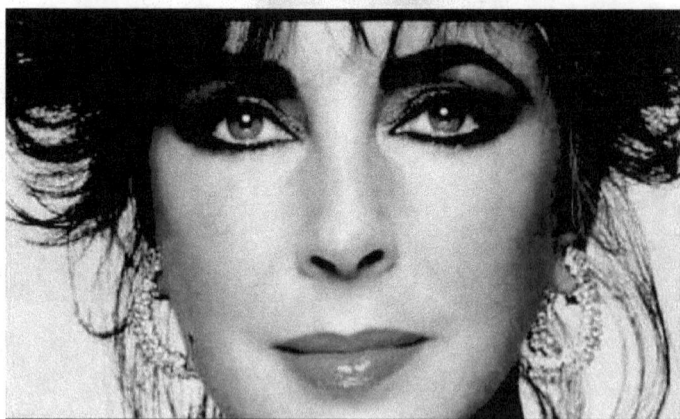

The eyes have it: Elizabeth Taylor has a long face. She was born with distichiasis, a genetic condition that resulted in an extra set of lashes

While the cause of the extra lashes is indeed a mutation - a result of an abnormal development of the FOXC2 gene - the effect of the luxurious lashes, also known as an 'accessory row', was entirely captivating, framing Taylor's deep violet eyes, and only adding to what admirers called her 'incandescent' beauty.

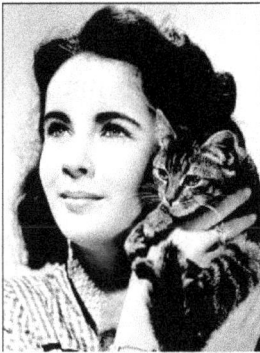

In her first film "Lassie" aged 9 in 1940, she was told she had too much eye makeup on but indeed was not wearing any. Would you ever change her eyebrow shape. No there is no need. Yes her brows are very thick and dark but they suit her violet coloured eyes. Elizabeth Taylor is a prime example of how eyebrows increase a woman beauty.

HOW OUR FACE AFFECTS OUR EYEBROWS

How our face affects the shape of your eyebrows. Certain parts of your face will impact the shape of your brows.

Everyone is unique, but we all have a flaw on our face that needs correcting. The correct colour and shape of our eyebrows will correct and take the focus away from our other flaws.

It could be:-

- The colour of our hair does not match the colour of our skin tone
- The size, width and length of our nose.
- The size of our eyes.
- The position of our nose in relation to our eyes.
- How our eyebrows naturally grow.

All of these aspects have an effect on the shape of our eyebrows.

FACE SHAPES.

In the Hairdressing, the Beauty industry and Optometry we have several face shapes to use as guides. The heart shaped face, the long, the square, the round. A long or square face maybe called a rectangular face. Many faces have a combination of these shapes. Skin colours and textures will also play a role in shaping eyebrows. However at the beginning of your beauty career or in deciding what your own personal eyebrow shape should be, to understand the basic face shapes is a wonderful tool.

WORKOUT A PERSONS FACE SHAPE.

Brush their hair back off the face and put a headband on their hair. Stand back and have a look. As time goes by you will find yourself looking at faces of people and working out what shape their brow should be to flatter their facial features.

The fashion of the century also plays a role. We also need to consider what the client is comfortable with. Let us think about this:-

If the client has darkish skin, with bleached blonde hair, a square face and bushy black eyebrows. You might suggest lightening the eyebrows then considering the shape. But the client may love their black eyebrows. In this case once you have assisted the client with the correct shape and they are happy with their new look you have a win, win situation.

This client will be back. After several visits and her trust in you have escalated, you may suggest you thin out the eyebrow a little.

Did you hear me.?

I said, a little.

Also, be very careful to inspect his or her brows before you make this suggestion. There are people that appear to have very thick eyebrows but on a closer inspection, you find they have long hairs but few of them or they may have a small bald patch hidden in there under long hairs. The least amount of change you make each session is often the best policy, with most clients.

Some clients will say yes, to everything you suggest and then go home and cry. They will tell all their friends how upset they are and never come back to your salon. Others will constantly allow you to do what you think should be done and keep coming back because they are loyal but may never be happy. Offer suggestion and be completely open with them. Help them to speak up for them self by designing your consultation to suit all personality types. You are there to please them not the other way around.

EYEBROW SHAPING FOR FACE SHAPES

Determining Your Face shape is very easy if you wrap a towel around your hair.

HEART FACE

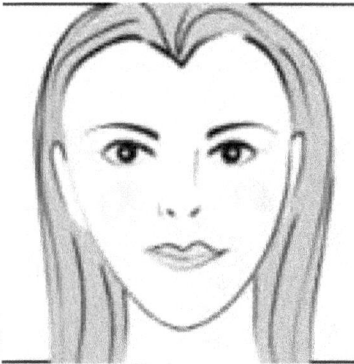

The upper half of face is broad, across the forehead and eyes, while the lower half narrows towards the chin.

• Add roundness to the shape of their brow to balance their narrow, pointed chin. You can achieve this by softening the peak of the arch with a pencil, or cosmetic tattooing.

• Keep the brows natural with a gentle arch; not too thick or thin.

LONG FACE

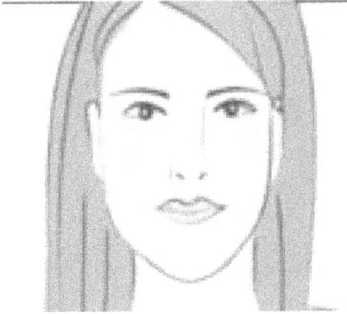

The jaw and cheekbones will be the same width and their chin may have a prominent shape. Create a wide brow by lengthening the ends with a pencil. These horizontal lines will draw the eye from side to side rather than up and down. A flat, arch-less brow will draw attention away from the length of their face and create the illusion of width. I would suggest that a feather fringe may also help especially if it sweeps to one side of the face.

Keep your brows thicker to add fullness to the face.

Elizabeth Taylor has thick eyebrows and always wears her hair in styles that have lots of curls and

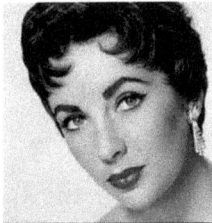

movement.

SQUARE FACE

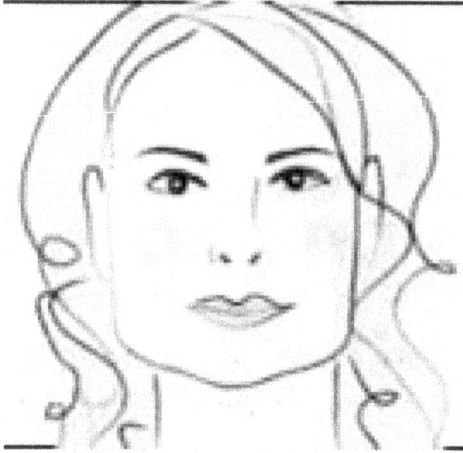

Their forehead, cheekbones and jaw will usually be an almost equal width and their jaw will be square. This face shape needs softening to avoid bone structure upstaging their features.

• Delicate, non-angular brows will accentuate the spatial placement of the eyes and create a facial balance.

• Eyebrows can be slightly thinner to soften their features.

ROUND FACE

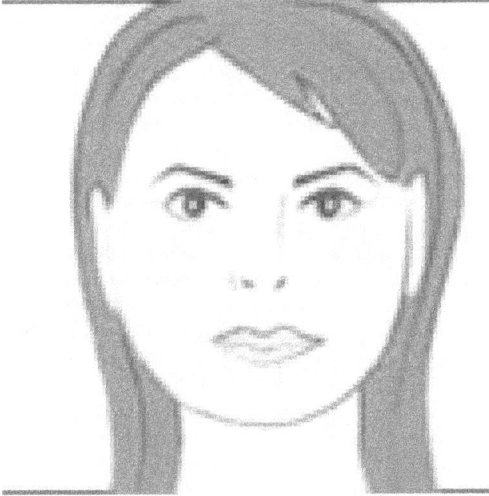

A round face is generally wide and may have a soft, circular shape without any prominent bone structure.

Angular brows will contrast this face shape and emphasise the eyes. Create a strong peak with an eyebrow pencil.

A high arch towards the end of the brow will balance the width of their face. To achieve this pluck the hairs below the arch to define the highest point with a brow pencil.

MY OPINION

Beautifully shaped brows make an amazing difference to a face. Changing the colour of the brows to enhance their hair colour should also be given enormous consideration.

However, grey or white hair should not be given grey or white eyebrows this ages the face. Take into account the colour of the skin and the skins undertones and colour the eyebrows accordingly. Try three or four different shades of brown eyeshadow on the brows before tinting them.

Take your time once you have given someone or yourself beautiful looking eyebrows great joy will be experienced. Great shaped brows add confidence to the personality of the person.

Everyone can pluck or wax eyebrows, but only a professional can shape eyebrows to enhance someone's beauty. Only a Beauty Therapist that truly loves her job will do an amazing reshaping of the eyebrows, so shop around.

If you are a Beauty Therapist reading this book, hopefully, you are one of those, who love her job and is passionate about the art of adorning others.

The first time you are looking for a more flattering brow shape. I strongly recommend you do not attempt to shape your own brows. Once the correct shape is there, you will be able to maintain them yourself.

The other point is that badly shaped eyebrow can take up to six months to repair and the older you become, the longer it will take to correct the shape. Therefore, it is best to stay with the one Beauty Therapist that you trust until your eyebrows become a flattering feature of your face.

There is a phenomenal difference, between the amounts of training Beauty Therapist receive at the different Beauty Schools. In my day Beauty Therapy Training was four years. These days they can obtain a Beauty Certificate in six to twelve weeks and a Diploma in six to twelve months. There are Therapist that thirst for knowledge and those that are in a rush to start earning money. You can tell the difference when you book to have your eyebrows done.

When a Therapist that thirsts for knowledge attends to your eyebrows she will clean the brow, brush the brow stand back and have a look at your face; she will then pencil in a shape, stand back and have another look. Give you a mirror and allow you to express your feelings. This unique Therapist is not trying to show you how good she is to gain a compliment she is genuinely concerned about how you feel.

This type of therapist may even pencil in a different shape on each eyebrow. Stand back and have a good look, hand you a mirror and discuss the different shapes and thickness with you and talk to you about eyebrow tinting or lightening. Another question will be what is your natural hair colour, how often do you change your hair colour and how long you intend to keep the hair colour you have right now.

DEFINE THE SHAPE.

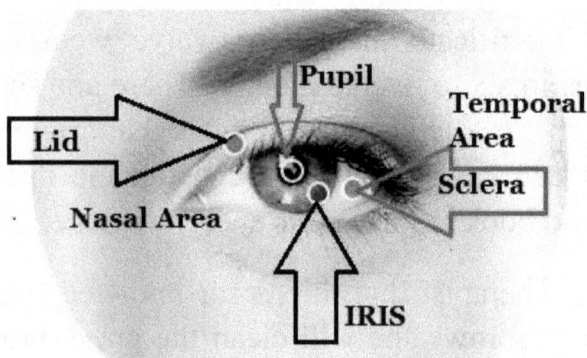

Pupil

Temporal Area

Lid

Sclera

Nasal Area

IRIS

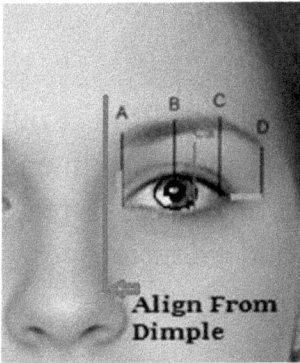

Align From
Dimple

Always take a conservative approach.
Never ever, remove more hair than is absolutely
required.

Before you start an eyebrow shaping process, you
must fully understand the best eyebrow shape for
your face shape. Please read the entire book before
you begin on clients and practice on family and
friends.

Please practice this on several family and friends
before you wax, pluck, thread or change anyone's
eyebrow shape.

When you measure, use callipers. Mark the spots
with a pencil designed for makeup use. You will need
several colours. If your friend has bushy eyebrows
use skin tone face paint to show the new shape, you
think would be best for them. Paint the face paint

onto the eyebrow area you think needs to be removed, from the eyebrow.

Another great way is to take a photo. Print it out in black and white and paint the section you intend to remove with white paint. This also works great for areas you may be intending to add extensions to.

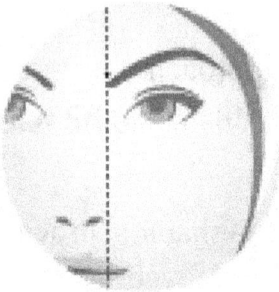

Always use the nose as the pivotal point to shape the eyebrows. For a thin nose, start at the outside of the nostril. For a broad nose start at the nose dimple

I like to use a tail comb or a bamboo stick.

In this section on how to define the shape, you need to understand that this is a guide and a general rule. Please consider the clients face shape before you begin these measurements and adjust these rules to the face shape.

1st   Sit the stick close to the nose to ascertain where the eyebrows should start. Note: if you or the client, have large nostrils and for a full nose, place the stick in line with the dimple in the nostril.

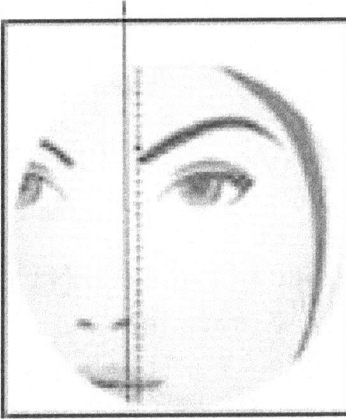

I myself have a wide nose so I also line up my position from my dimple in my nostril. To decrease the size of my nose I also put a little brown eye shadow on the side of my nose after I have finished putting my makeup on. Blend the eyebrow eye-shadow powder in well to the side of the nose so it is just a shadow that can barely be seen. This technique gives a slimmer look to your nose as well as a more flattering look to your eyebrows.

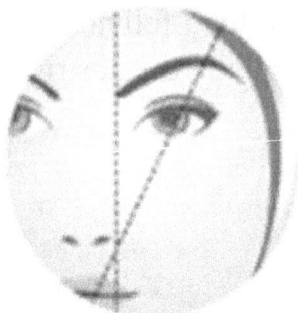

2nd. Sit the stick on the side of the nose. Have the client look straight ahead now move the stick in line with the outside of the Pupil. This is a line that is very hard to attend to yourself as you will be looking at the line and may not have your eyes in the correct position. This line gives the correct position for the arch. For a wide nose use the same point as explained above in the first explanation.

Remember if they have a very wide nose take the line from their nostril not the side of the nose. You may find with this line will end with the same result from both starting points.

3rd. Again sit the stick at the edge of the nose. Look straight ahead and line the stick with the outside edge of the skin at the endpoint of the eye. This is where the eyebrow should finish. For a wide nose use the same point as explained above in 1st explanation.

However, in the second photo on page 42 I like to use the "C" point for this measurement.

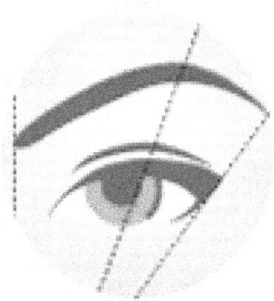

For people with close-set eyes, the gap between the brows should be left wider. For clients, whose eyes are far apart; the gap should be less. This creates balanceing illusion. Be careful to adjust if they have a wide nose.

To calculate the curve and mark the highest point of the brow arch, hold the ruler from the edge of the nostril past the outer edge of the iris up to the eyebrow and mark it with a dot too. Link the dots in a gentle smooth arch that slightly tapers at the outer ends.

MEASURE THE FACE AND EYEBROWS.

When you measure the face with callipers you will be enlightened.

First find the centre of the face and place a small mark.

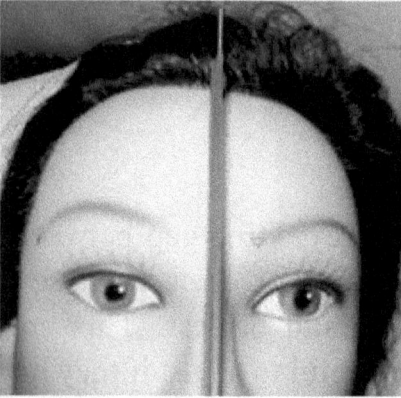

Next measure end to end of the eyebrows and place a small mark.

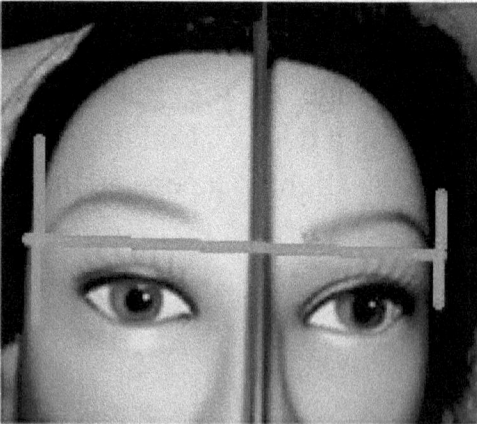

Find the centre of each brow. The client should be looking straight ahead. The centre will differ on all clients depending on the width of their nose and the set position of their eyes. Notice my dolls eyes are a bit wacko and the same may be with your client. If so you will need to make some adjustments to suit.

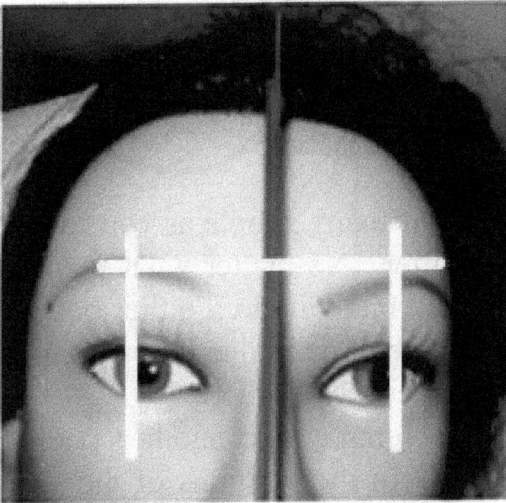

Next, measure the width of each eyebrow and place small marks. From Nose centre to arch centre. Then the nose centre to outer edge of the brow.

Eyebrow Shaping & Colouring To Suit Face Shapes

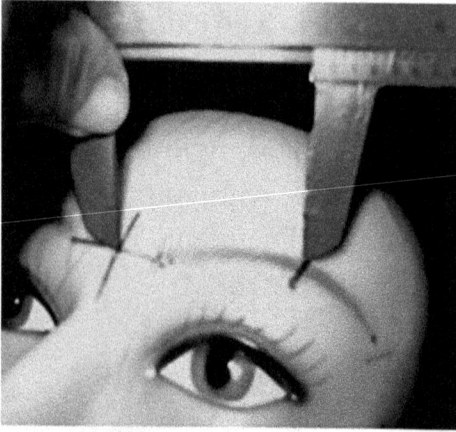

Try this exercise on as many people as you can. Take photos before and after. No matter what shape their eyebrows are; try to create an arch either pointed or curved depending on their natural eyebrow shape.

Only create a slight arch. Take another photo and access your study. Gain the opinions of the subjects (people) it is important to note how they feel about the position and shape of their arch. It is also best to find people that have not attended to their eyebrows for the last six or more weeks. You must first tell them it is an eyebrow shaping study.

Whenever I was training a new apprentice, I would put a board outside my salon for three weeks before the study.

The sign would say:-

Free Eye Enhancement
To anyone that will take part in our Eyebrow to suit
face shape study.
Dates ....
Times ....
Help our apprentice to become great and book in
today.
Put Apprentice Name Here........
Will be guided by
Put Salon Owner Name here ....

Then I would have a small eye enhancement
brochure to give them.

Failing this opportunity, you can invite family,
acquaintances and friends to assist you with your
study.

HAIR STYLES AND HAIR COLOUR

DARK HAIR

How you or your client wear your hair will also play a vital role in how the eyebrows should be shaped. If the hair is thick and dark and wear off the face the eyebrows should be a dash thinner and slightly more curved at the arch than if this same hairstyle type were to have a fringe. When the hair is dark and thick, and you have a fringe, then extra attention must be given to the sharpness of the arch. When their skin is pale, their eyebrows should be lightened, even though they have very dark hair. When the hair is very fine and they have dark hair that they wear is a fluffy curly style soften their eyebrows but give them a sharp over defined arch.

REDHEADS

red Heads need softly shaped brows without a point no matter what their hairstyle or face shape. However, there are always, an exception to the rule.

BLONDE HAIR

A blonde should never engage in the thought of black or dark brown eyebrows. No matter what type of hairstyle they have. Their eyebrows will look better coloured in a light brown or taupe. This rule applies even if the client has dark skin and once had dark hair.

GREY HAIR

Should never leave their eyebrows a grey, black or dark brown shade, no matter what their hairstyle or skin tone is. Taupe looks best as a colour for all hairstyles and face shape.

BEST STYLES ON A HEART-SHAPED FACE

Heart-shaped faces are wider at the forehead and gently narrow down at the jaw line. Your chin may even be somewhat adoringly pointy. Watch how Reese Witherspoon and Katie Holmes wear their hair. This shape is also known as the "inverted-triangle."

Short pixie style haircuts work well for heart shaped faces. Your cute pointy chin tends to be the focal point of your face. Draw attention to your eyes and cheekbones with side-swept bangs. Allow your fringe to feather sideways over one of your eyebrows. Flick your hair back over your ears. Or style your hair in an up-style with a flicking sideway fringe. Have a strong part and hair that falls at or below your jaw line. Keep top layers soft and feathering. If you like long hair, go for long layers that feather onto your cheekbones.

BEST STYLES ON A SQUARE FACE

Photographers claim that square faces photograph the best. A square face is a face that the width of forehead, cheekbones, and jaw are almost equal in width, with sharp angular features including a sharp jaw line. A square face, needs to consider styles that also suit famous faces in the past and today such as , Demi Moore and Keira Knightley.

They have a strong, attractive angular jaw line.

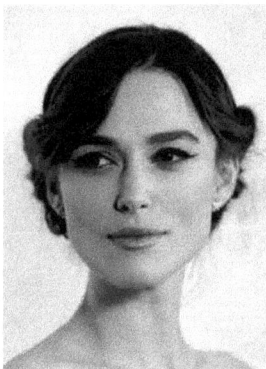

Keira Knightley

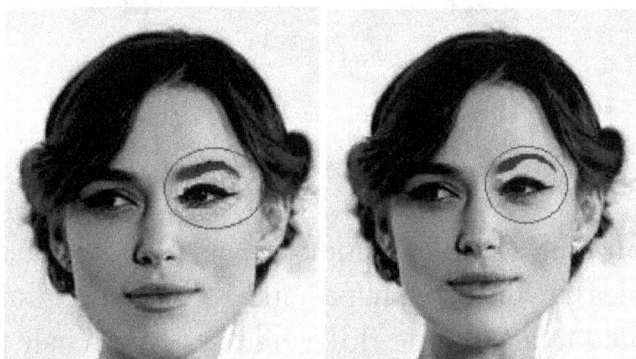

Although my art work is lousy, it is easy to tell Keira needs a more flattering shape to her eyebrows. In the photo on the left, I have given her a peaked brow and the on the right an arched brow. The arch brow lifts her face where the peak brow softens her jaw line. She is very beautiful, but a softer brow shape would give her an automatic lift in the eye area. Especially, when she is tired or starting to age.

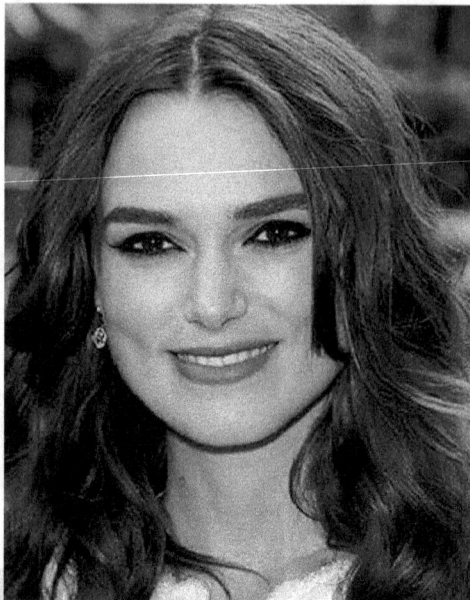

However, in this section we are talking about hair styles to suit face shapes and Keira is definitely well suited to a full long fluffy hair style with hair flowing around her chin line. When wearing her hair in an up-style Keira needs little wispy bits of hair around the nape of her neck.

In the next Photo of the very attractive Demi Moore You will notice how a long straight hair style does not do her justice. Her peak in her eyebrow is also t sudden and sharp.

Both these issues accentuate her jaw line and pronounce it as wide.

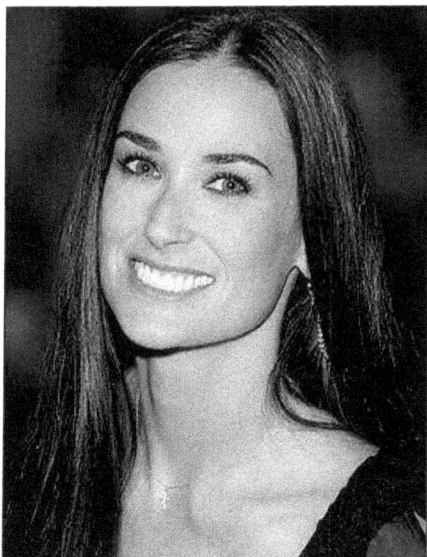

Demi Moore has a combination shape face, Square Oblong.

When Demi Moore wears her hair hanging straight down the front, she looks tired.

Demi is at her loveliest when her hair is flowing in long wavy styles. I think she looks too stiff when her hair is in up styles unless it has soft wisps, hanging out. That is when her face says to us I am a lovely

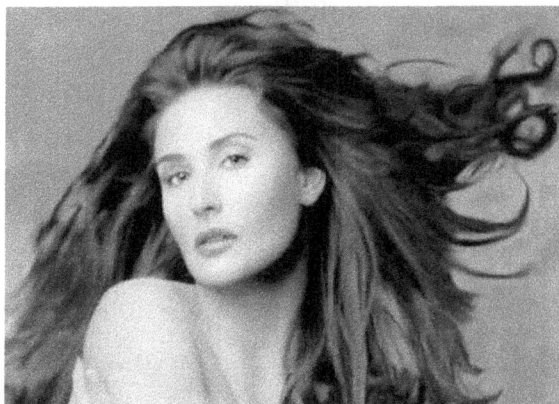

person. I am approachable.

The same would have to be said about Keira Knightly

If you have a square face, you may want to play down your strong, angular jaw. Texture, type of hair styles with formed curls or choppy ends works brilliantly. You can also get away with short, spiky cuts and long, sleek styles with layers that start at the jaw line and continue downward. A whipped fringe and up-styles look great on this face shape as well.

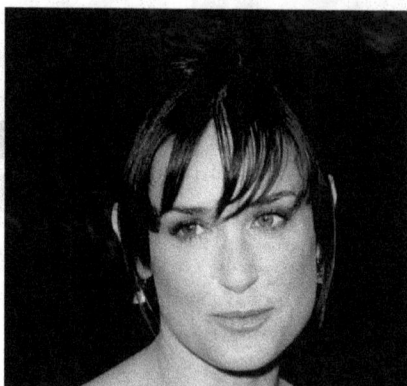

The books I read when I was young suggested, long bobs are an excellent choice. However, bobs are not flattering, and you need to be very careful when choosing the length of the bob. Avoid one-length bob hairstyles especially chin-length with wide, blunt lengths. These will only highlight your angular features rather than downplay them.

Side-swept styles or hair flowing gently to one side of the face will beautify your face shape. A geometric cut with one side cut up around the ear and the other side long, looks great on a square face. Celebrities with a square shaped face **Gwyneth Paltrow, Demi Moore** and **Angelina Jolie** and **Keira Knightly.**

BEST STYLES ON A ROUND FACE

A round face will have a width of forehead, cheekbones, and jawline that will probably be an equal width that will say hello to others looking at this face. The jaw is slightly rounded as opposed to angular with soft features. Square faces have strong, angular features, whereas a round face has soft features and full cheekbones.

Round faces tend to be soft with non-angular features and full cheeks. You may find you have more of a round face when you carry extra weight, but keep in mind many classic round-faced women are super thin and still have non-angular features.

Typically, if you have a round face, you want to make your face appear longer, leaner and less round. To do this, create less volume around the face. A longer style that falls below the chin line with soft, graduated layers are best, because they will make your face appear slimmer and tend to remove bulk and weight from the sides. Consider long wispy and tapered ends with a side sweep. like Rihanna. Famous people that share your face shape are;- Duchess Fergie, Oprah Winfrey, Cameron Diaz, Kirsten Dunst, Catherine Zeta-Jones.

Avoid one-length, blunt cuts such as the classic bob hairstyle if you have short hair. Curly, short hair is also a no-no. Grow your curls out to shoulder-length.

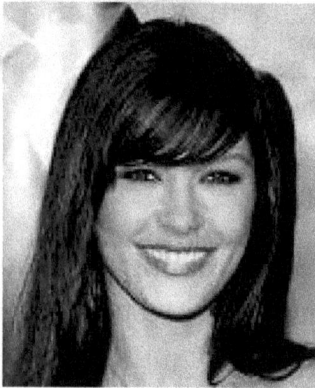

When Catherine Zeta-Jones Wears her hair down her face looks more heart shaped. With an up style her face looks more round. This is not a problem with her beautiful face. However, she looks sexier with her hair long and flowing and more debonair with it up.

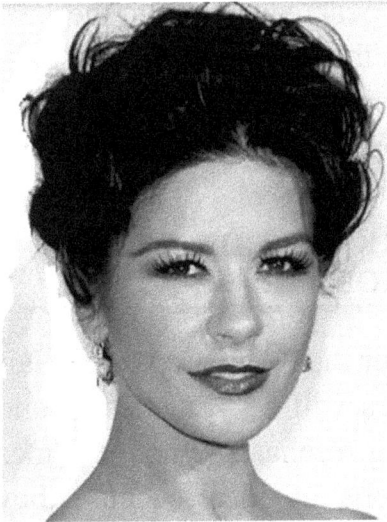

Her eyebrow shape is also peaked and that is perfect for her face shape.

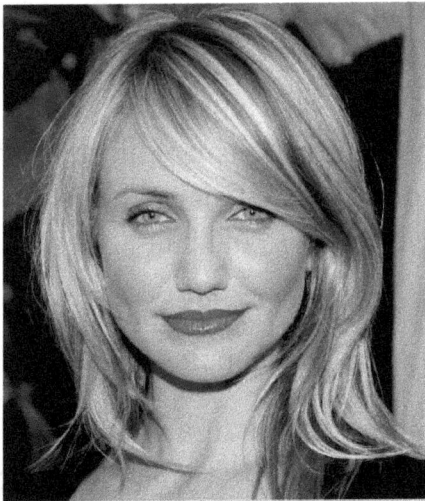

Cameron Diaz

In this photo her eyebrow peak is way out to the outer boundary of her eyes this does widen her look and she needs that as she is very slim. As she ages her brow peak will need to come inward a dash more.

STYLES THAT WORK BEST ON A LONG FACE

Long face shapes are longer than they are wide. Hair that flips our from the ears will be your best friend because they can hide a big forehead. When it comes to haircuts, chin-length bobs are ideal because they create the illusion of width. Gwyneth Paltrows long bob is very flattering on a long face. Just make sure your stylist cuts the hair a bit shorter in the back. Curls and waves work well because they add width to the face. Long hair that is too long can drag down the face. Long layers work best with pieces hitting at the nose, the chin and the collarbone. Consider a v-shaped style where the length is mainly in the back, while the sides and front of your hair appear shorter. Consider adding wave or curls to the hair style.

Stay away from the extremes. Don't go longer than the collarbone and avoid a skull-capping pixie cut.

Cate Blanchet is a prime example of a women with a long face and clearly Cate looks best when her hair is fluffed out around the jaw line. Her eyebrow tint is a perfect colour for her hair colour and skin type. Note each of her eyebrows are a slightly different shape and thickness. This could be made less obvious by applying the eyebrow tint to her left eyebrow for five to ten minutes longer than her right side. However it could be the lighting in the room when this photo was taken. The lesson here is to know that we are not perfectly symmetrical.

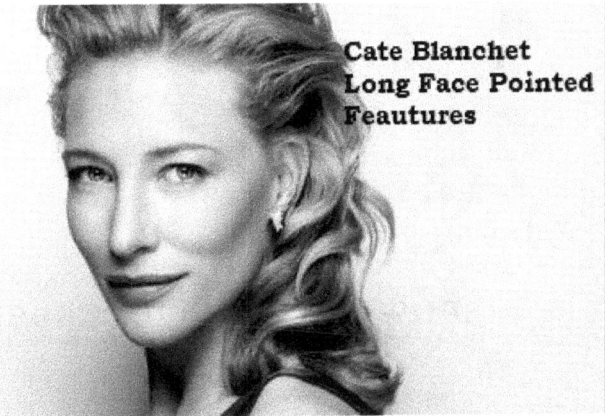

Cate Blanchet
Long Face Pointed
Feautures

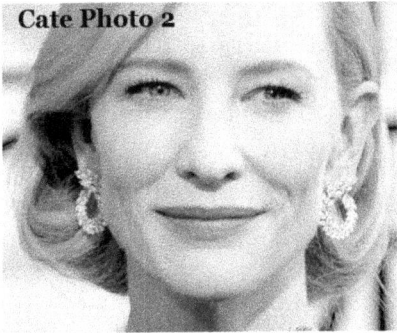

Cate Photo 2

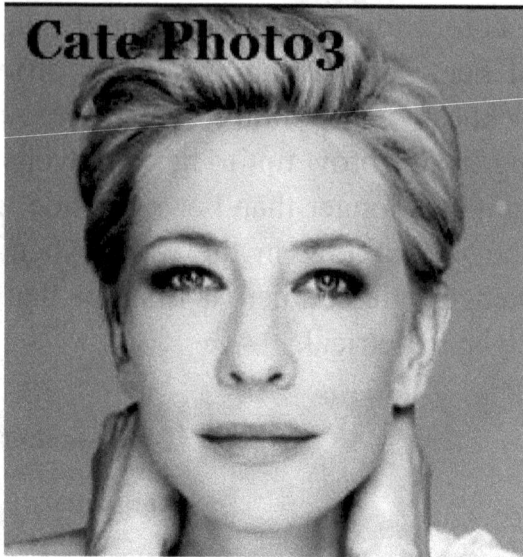

EYEBROW SHAPING PROCEDURE.

Providing your client is not sunburned nor on any strong medication and you have filled in your client form and had her sign the form you can begin.

With all that you have learned about shaping to suit face shapes and the test you have been doing on friends and family you should be ready to consult with your client.

Once you have decided on their eyebrow shape and colour, you can begin.

1. Clean and prepare the eyebrow skin. Use a gentle cleanser and remove it. Then place some toner on a pad and tone the skin. Be very gentle you do not want to bring too much blood to the skin surface, as when the hot wax is applied it will burn the skin because you warmed the skin too much.

2. Apply astringent on the brow area to clean and make it numb for a short time.

3. Before waxing the brows, it is important to prepare them beforehand using an eye brush to define their natural shape. See instruction above for "defining the shape."

4. Trim very long hairs. But first, be sure that if you trim it is not going to expose a small bald patch in the eyebrow.

5..Calculate the length of the eyebrow the client wants and needs. Holding a stick parallel to their nose, levelling it with the inner corner of the eye to see where the brow should begin and mark the point with a dot using the brow pencil.

6...Apply the pre-wax oil with a cotton pad.

7...Apply wax on half of each eyebrow.

8...Press the wax into the skin.

9...Put a small dab of wax on your thumb. With one hand pull the skin tight. With the other hand remove the wax by putting the waxed thumb onto the wax corner and pull along the eyebrow towards the nose. Repeat this procedure on the other eyebrow.

10...Firmly press your finger pads on the eyebrows where you have just removed the wax from.

11...Apply wax to the other half of the eyebrows. Repeat steps 8, 9. and 10.

12...Apply a cold cloth to the brows and press firm for one minute.

13...Now check the shape and only re-wax if you need to. You may need to use the tweezers to remove a hair or two in the arch.

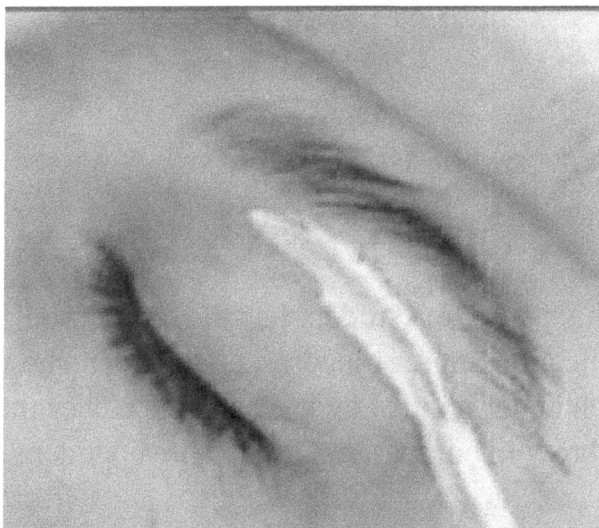

Note: How the wax is applied to lower than the brow shape. You then push the wax up into the curve. I think this student has positioned her wax reasonably well but is using the wrong type of applicator and has started the wax position too far to the left. The wax has gone the full length of the brow. It is best to use a wax stick. With an eyebrow timber stick you can gather a lot of wax on the tip of the stick and at a 45-degree angle get a better shape with the wax.

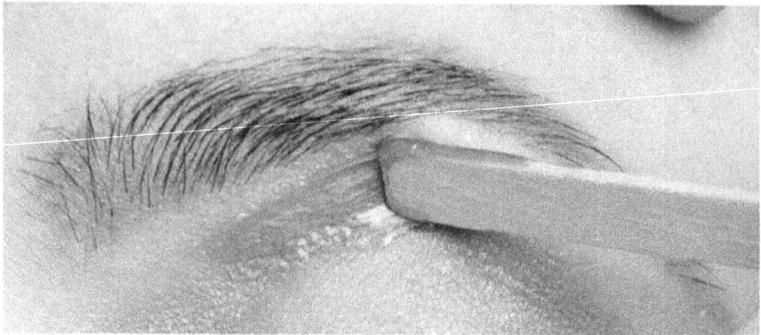

In this photo, the student has the correct tool, but her application angle is incorrect. However, she will have much better control over where she places the wax on the brow in comparison to the above student.

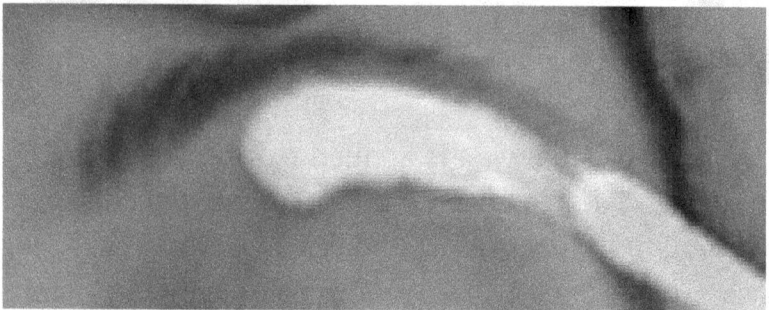

This photo shows the student has applied the wax at the correct angle and applied a good thick amount of wax. However, this student has allowed the wax to thin out at the outer edge. It is important for it to be thicker on the outer edge. She has applied in a curved motion which is excellent and has applied wax to just half of the area while holding and pulling the eyebrow skin firmly up toward the hairline. I would give this student 90% for this application.

Never apply the wax in one long strip like the photo below.

This will cause to much stress on the delicate eye skin as you pull it off. It will also cause some hair to break as you pull off.

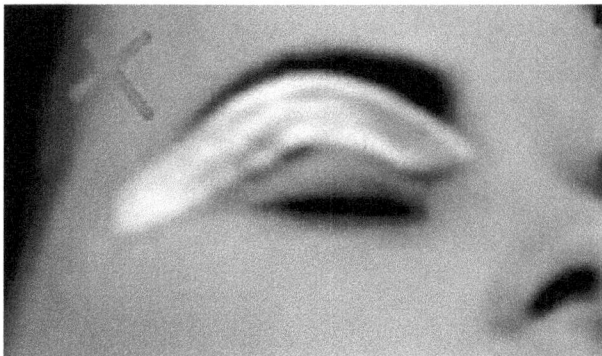

CLEAN AND PREPARE THE EYEBROW SKIN EXPLAINED FURTHER.

Apply astringent on the brow area to clean and make it numb for some time. The mixture I make and use is very simple to make at home or in your salon. Buy some witch hazel from the chemist or pharmacy.

MAKE ASTRINGENT /TONER

In a clean dark glass bottle pour 40 ml of witch hazel.

Add 60 ml of distilled or boiled water.

The water must be boiled for at least ten minutes then allowed to cool down.

Add 5 drops of Rose Geranium.

Shake well and allow to sit in a cool dark place for a few days before using this mix.

Pour a little of the mix onto a cotton-wool pad and apply to the eyebrows this mix will clean and numb the eyebrows.

PREPARING BROWS BRIEF

Before waxing the brows, it is important to prepare them beforehand using a eye brush to define their natural shape. Bush them in their shape then have a look. Now brush them up towards the forehead and trim the ones that are too long.

Calculate the length of the eyebrow the client wants and needs. Holding a stick parallel to their nose, levelling it with the inner corner of the eye to see where the brow should begin and mark the point with a dot using the brow pencil. Or hold on the nostril for larger noses.

For people with close-set eyes, the gap between the brows, should be left wider while those whose eyes are far apart; the gap should be less for a balancing illusion. Be careful to adjust if they have a wide nose.

To calculate the curve and mark the highest point of the brow arch, hold the ruler from the edge of the nostril past the outer edge of the iris up to the eyebrow and mark it with a dot too.

Link the dots in a gentle, smooth arch that slightly tapers at the outer ends. Consider in some eyebrow shapes the tip many need lifting slightly. You may need to remove some of the outer tip and colour above their natural shape.

An Eyebrow brush with a comb is a must have. It is important to brush straight up then comb up and snip above the comb. Be mindful of long hairs that are covering bald spots.

Eyebrow powders give a soft appearance eyebrow pencils give definition.

Use two or three shade for a more natural look.

My three favourite eyebrow brushes.

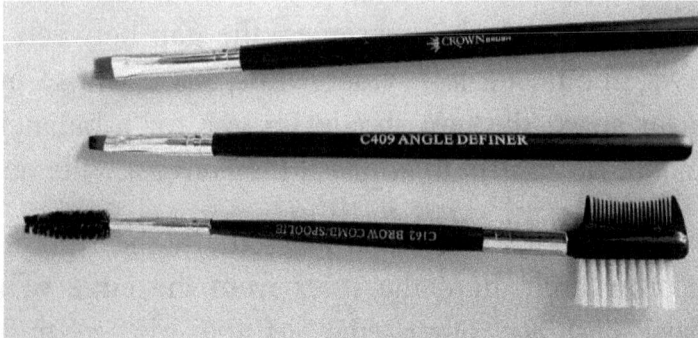

From, http://www.crownbrush.com.au/products/luna-series

WAX TYPES

HOT WAX

Hot wax is a gentle wax when at the right temperature and does not need to be taken off with a cotton strip. You press it on and pull it off with your fingers or the spatula. It usually has fruit oils added. This is by far the best wax and waxing method for facial and sphinx waxing.

Such as:-

- eyebrows

- lip wax

- chin

- ear lobes

- nostrils

- blackhead removal

- the centre of virginal

- inner posterior (buttocks)

HOT WAX POT.

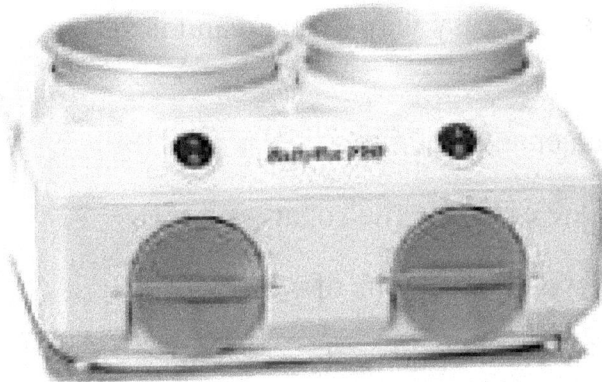

Hot Wax is by far the best wax for all facial waxing procedures. I have included the other types of waxes Therapist use in the Salon.

It is funny that they call this gentle wax "HOT WAX" as it is applied less hot than the strip wax. It is also applied very thick and is more expensive than strip wax. Hot wax is the correct type of wax for all facial waxing procedures. There is much more about waxing in my book called:-

"Body & Face Waxing Cosmetology Hair Removal."

However, for eyebrow waxing, this is the only wax you need to know about. Apricot wax is by far my favourite wax. Next is Sugar wax and I have included a recipe here for Sugar wax.

SUGAR WAX

This is a very easy wax to make and is very gentle on the skin.

To a saucepan add

1. One cup of white sugar

2. Two tablespoons of water

3. Two tablespoons of lemon juice.

4. Over a low heat stir for about five minutes until the sugar mixture changes to an amber or ginger ale colour.

5. When you turn the heat off wait a few minutes . Then add 2 drops of essential oil of Rose Geranium.

6. Place in a metal wax pot or glass jar.

7. Allow to cool a little and apply the same way as hot wax.

I make it in my Hot Wax Pot as pictured above. You can use raw or brown sugar but try it with white sugar a few times first until you become familiar with the colour change and how long it takes you to melt the sugar.

You can also turn this into a strip wax by adding two more tablespoons of water.

TEST THE WAX HEAT

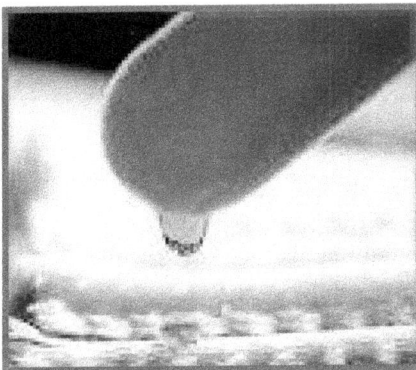

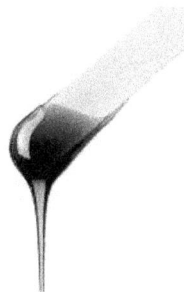

In both the above pictures, the wax is too hot.

If it drops in a thin flow, it is too hot.

Before I talk about wax types I want you to note if the wax is dripping off the applicator as it is in this photo, then the wax is far too hot. Always test it over the wax pot first. If the wax drips easily or runs off the applicator, turn the wax off for a couple of minutes. Then recheck it by dipping a new stick into the pot. If it is thick and slow to come off the applicator, then it is possibly ready. Now dip the applicator into the pot and place a small amount onto your own wrist.

STRIP WAX POT

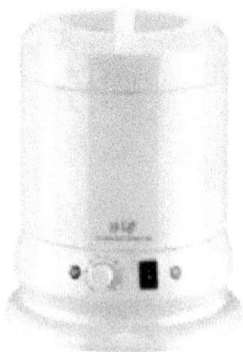

Strip Wax is usually heated in a larger pot. Applied with a wood spatula and removed with strips of cloth. Strip wax should never ever be used on the face no matter what any supplier tells you.

ROLLER WAX

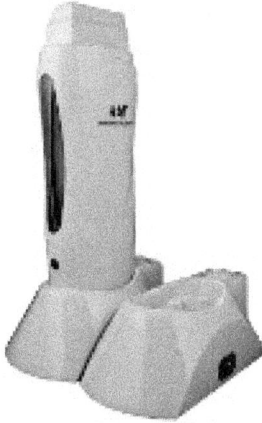

Never ever use a roller wax on the face even though the suppliers produce a tiny roller for the face. However after 50 plus years in a salon I stress do not use this wax for eyebrows. This wax is to be used on the body, not on the face. This is by far my favourite type of wax for body waxing but never ever use on long hair. You should trim hair first.

Roller wax is for body waxing only and is not suitable for eyebrow waxing. They do come with a mini head that is designed for eyebrows, but I strongly recommend you do not use it. Shaping eyebrows correctly with the mini roller head is almost impossible. They do not roll to the right shape for the brow.

ROLLER WAX INSERT.

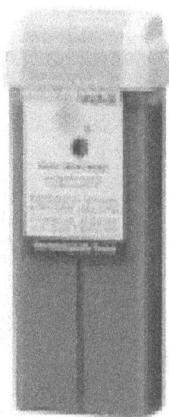

The Australian Standards requires for health and hygiene reasons that you use this roller wax insert on one client only. This makes it expensive unless you have a cupboard to keep each client left over wax.

A PROFESSIONAL WAXING KIT.

All types of wax pots and rollers have a temperature control button. See manufactures instructions. All types of wax have their own procedures. Hot wax usually requires an oil base applied to the eyebrow before applying the wax, or it will not work. Most strip waxes require a talc applied to the skin or they will not work. Talc should never ever be used on clients face no matter how careful you are. That is why I advocate hot wax methods for eyebrow shaping.

Naturally, you will need a professional waxing kit for shaping eyebrows.

EYEBROW HOT WAX KIT

1. Camera

2. Eyebrow brush. Clean with alcohol before and after use.

3. Eyebrow pencil. Clean with alcohol wipes.

4. Eyebrow scissors. They must be sterilized and in the autoclave bag.

5. Tweezers in sterilized autoclave pack.

6. A temperature controlled wax pot.

7. Wax. *I like apricot wax.*

8. Wooden single use spatulas in a few sizes

9. Astringent. To clean skin

10. Oil to apply before the wax (but see wax manufacturers instruction)

11. Icy cold face cloth. *To apply with pressure after the wax.*

12. Gauze pads to apply the lotions and dry the eyebrows.

13. A soothing oil or cream for after the application

14. Alcohol for cleaning brushes and tweezers.

15. Alcohol wipes for cleaning pencil. Never use alcohol on clients skin after a procedure and be sure the client is not allergic to alcohol before the procedure.

16. Never ever use Talc on a clients face.

APPLY AND REMOVE HOT WAX

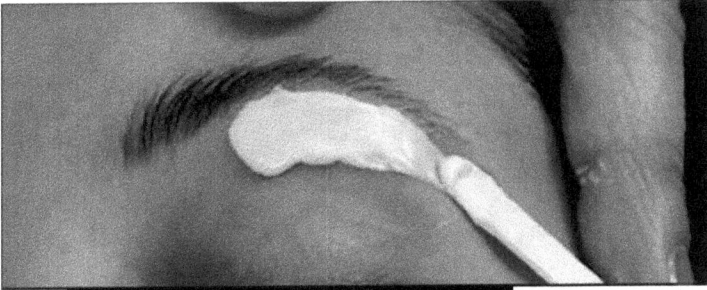

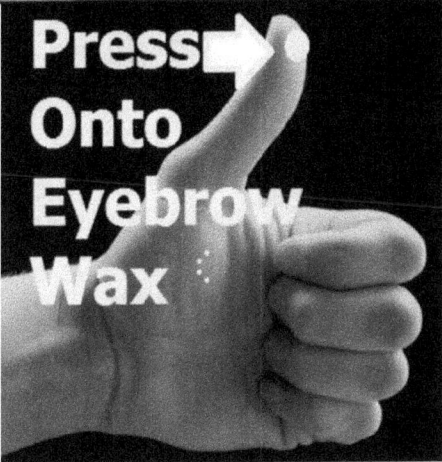

Design the eyebrows first show the shape to the client with a pencil.

* Warm the wax to an optimum temperature. If you do not have a commercial wax pot, you can warm the wax in the microwave and keep the jar sitting in a pot of boiling water and then use the spatula to apply a thin layer of wax on the stray hairs under the eyebrow in the direction of the hair growth.

APPLY AND REMOVE HOT WAX

- Warm wax to the optimum temperature.

- Test Wax heat on your wrist.

- Apply in the correct shape.

- For hot wax you remove by pressing down on the wax and pulling off with your fingers. Or

- Remove eyebrow wax by placing a small ball of wax onto your thumb tip. Place your thumb tip on the outer edge of the wax you applied to the underside of the brow. Press down. Use your other hand to stretch the skin.

- Pull wax off in the opposite direction of the hair growth as directed on the kit before the wax dries.

- Be certain that you have placed you fingers each side of the wax to hold the skin tightly stretched.

- You can also place a small amount of wax on the stick (a spatula} place that on the tip of the outside edge of the wax to remove the wax.

- When you use your fingernail to lift the end of the wax it hurts.

- For those of you intending to do the professional course, the right technique will be demonstrated. Each manufacturer has their own instruction sheet be sure to obtain one before using their wax.

- Never wax above the eyebrows. Unless absolutely necessary.

- For thick growth, it is better and less painful to wax off a little hair at the time.

- For thin eyebrows less is best. Keep the eyebrows a little thicker in height. This type of client will benefit from both eyebrow tinting and eyebrow tattooing.

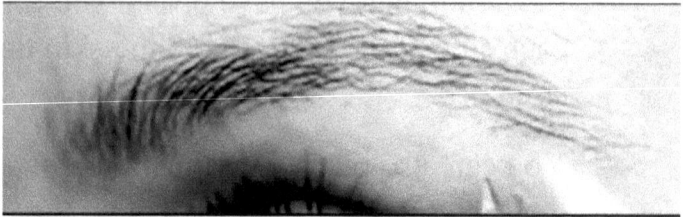

- Pluck any stray hair using a set of good tweezers and apply a soothing balm on the area.

- Be careful enough to avoid direct sunlight, acid based facial treatments and liquid makeup for some hours after an eyebrow wax.

- Emphasise your brows using an eyebrow pencil or tinted brow shadow.

- Take to class photos of family members and friends eyebrows that need shaping. Your teacher will give you ideas on how to shape each person brows.

EYEBROW SHAPING BRIEF.

- Define shape

- Clean Brows

- Brush and trim

- Oil on and wipe off. (see manufacturers sheet)

- Apply warm not hot wax to half the brow

- Press down on wax

- Hold the outer edge of the eye very firm

- Lift and pull off from outer edge towards nose, never lift wax up

- Pat their brow firmly this will reduce the pain

- Apply warm not hot wax to the other half of the eyebrow

- Press down on wax

- Lift and pull off from outer edge towards the nose, never lift wax up

- Pat their brow firmly this will reduce the pain

- Repeat these step on the other eyebrow

- Clean the eyebrows and apply a cold face cloth with pressure.

- Use tweezers on stray hairs there should only be a few.

Before you trim watch for bald patches in the eyebrow area. Some people have long hairs that cover that bald spot. When you brush down and trim, you can expose those bald spots. When I was young, I made that mistake a few times.

HAIR THREADING TECHNIQUE

I love threading; it is one of the best eyebrow hair removal techniques. You can thread your legs or almost any part of your body, and I strongly suggest you practice on your leg before trying someones eyebrows.

You cannot learn to thread from a book or anyone just explaining what to do. You need to be shown, and you need to practice over and over.

Unlike waxing, where you can read the instructions and every time you do it you get better. Threading can tear delicate skin tissue and leave a blood red mark or worse. Threading does grab the hair at the root and it does hurt. it also gives a cleaner smoother look when done right and the hair will take three times longer to grow back.

If tweezers give your client the willies and waxing sounds cruel or they have very sensitive skin, then threading will most definitely be the hair removal technique for your client. See what happens when hair is threaded on YouTube videos.

Warning: If your client is mature age threading is most definitely a big no no. Their skin moves, and no matter how tight they pull on their brow to assist you, you will gather skin in the cotton, and it will tear.

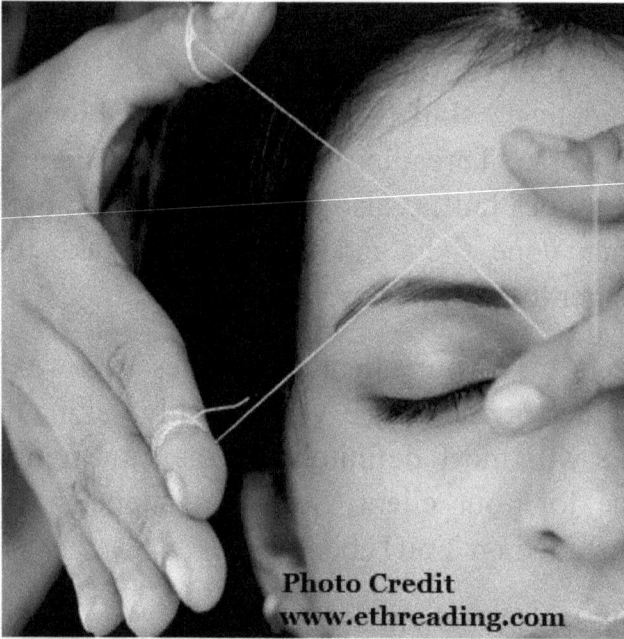

Photo Credit
www.ethreading.com

Threading Eyebrows Photo

Compliments of E-Threading

Watch some You- tube sites on how to do this and practice on young friends. Never ever perform threading on mature skin types.

EYEBROW TINTING KIT

A typical eyebrow tinting kit consists of:-

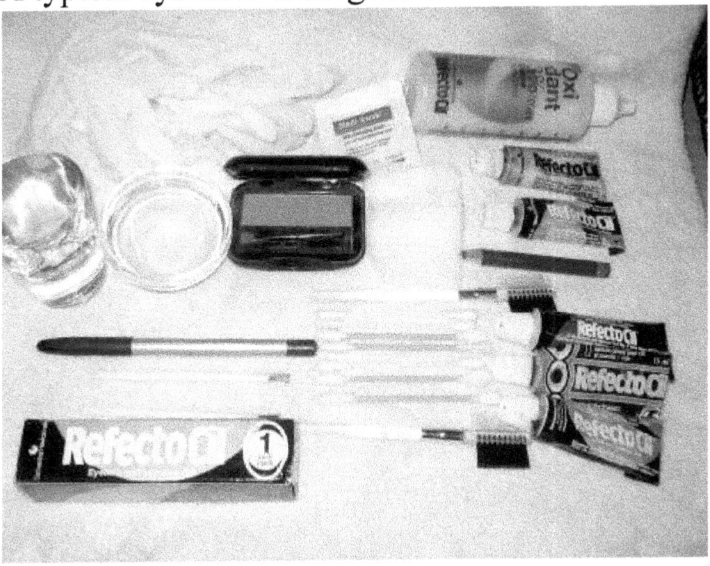

- Peroxide 3%

- Tint

- Gloves

- Eyebrow pencil

- Eyebrow powder

- Scissors

- Gloves

- Alcohol wipes

- Brush
- Cotton tips with pointed tips
- Cotton pads
- Gauze pads
- Glass mixing bowl
- Applicator
- Alcohol in a Glass mug.
- Cleanser and toner.
- Ice pack and face cloth

BEFORE YOU TINT BROWS OR LASHES.

You will notice here I constantly refer to Reflect- Cil it was easier to write this information with a product in mind. I myself, as you can see from the above photo have used their products for longer than I can remember so I know it well. This does not mean that you should use this product. You are you, and I am I. There are other great products in your salon supply stores but, be sure you know their product well before using it and be sure they supply mixing instruction with colour there notes.

Most of the suppliers say to leave the eyebrow tint on for ten minutes. I have found that it lasts longer if it is on for about 45 minutes. However, most clients do not have that amount of time. You need to plan their treatment and encourage them to have another treatment so they are there longer.

With my regular eye enhancement clients that are not having any other treatments, I would encourage them to have a twenty minutes hand and foot mask. I would always offer them this treatment at half price. Apply their eyelash and eyebrow tint then apply their hand and foot mask.

Should they not want a foot and hand mask at least place a massage pad under their back. When a client is feeling relaxed, they are more inclined to lay there longer.

This gives the eyebrow tint more time to take. The longer the eyebrow tint lasts, the happier the client will be with your service.

A PATCH TEST INFORMATION

A patch test will be necessary. There are a small number of individuals, who may have an allergic reaction to tints, hair dyes and other chemical treatments. It is only in rare situations that the reaction can be severe.

The comfort of the client is essential to eliminate any discomfort. The health authorities and your insurance company require you to perform a test patch on all new clients. It is also advisable to do a test patch on older clients that have not had treatment for a while. Even people who have their eyelashes and eyebrows tinted regularly can still have an allergic reaction. If the client refuses to have this test, it is worthwhile having a salon policy, that the customer would have to sign a waiver. Please read carefully the instructions on how to perform a skin sensitivity test, which is included with every tint. I have this on their client card. Point it out to them at least once a year.

DANGERS OF VASELINE & BARRIER CREAMS

Never ever use Vaseline or a barrier cream on a clients face. I do not care what you were taught at Beauty school. Only the use of Refectocil Skin Protection Cream should be used around the eyes as it has been specially developed for the sensitive eye area. Or if you have been trained to use essential oils use Chamomile diluted in Jojoba oil (pronounced Ho-ho-ba}. In the "PAST" many other products were used to provide a barrier and protection from staining the skin. However with constant research, it was discovered that it was these kinds of products which caused reactions to the delicate skin around the eyes, not the tinting process itself.

Pregnant women should NOT be advised to have any chemical treatment unless it is their choice to do so. Each individual is different and again if they choose to proceed with the treatment the skin sensitivity/patch test MUST be performed at least 24 hours before the treatment. It is an absolute must that all salon operators have a treatment risk and salon policy form, each client should complete and sign. So every treatment is explained, and you have made your client aware of your salon's policies and the possible dangers.

There are approximately 10 different colour shades for tinting eyelashes and eyebrows or for lightening eyebrows. Before tinting consult, with the client about their wishes and expectations. The tint companies like Refectocil have a Colour Chart you can easily show, which tinting results can be achieved from the different colour shades. Some shades are suitable for every natural hair colour (pure black, blue-black, natural brown, chestnut, red, blonde); other shades are suitable only for lighter natural hair colours (deep blue, graphite, light brown, purple). On the colour-chart no colour result is indicated for unsuitable combinations.

The correct position for the client during tinting is not lying down, sitting and/or slightly leaning back is not suitable. The eyes must remain closed during tinting. The client should relax, direct the gaze downward or straight ahead, and not move the eyes.

If it is difficult for your client to keep the eyes still during the application time of the lash tint place a dampened cotton pad on each of the closed eyelids; this makes it easier to keep eyes closed. Be sure the pad is barely moistened and be sure it does not touch the eyelashes. I always tape the pad to the skin so it is less likely to move.

The coloring of hair, eyebrows and lashes was for a long time the sole domain of the woman, cross dressers, and male dancers. But with the consistently rising number of men, who attach particular importance to personal care, men have discovered the incomparable advantages of eyelash and eyebrow tints: to look simply better with longer and more voluminous lashes and brows. Lasting up to 4 weeks! people with fine hair or dry hair their tint may only last a week or so.

With an eyelash and eyebrow tint, men can finally give themselves a little "help", in order to emphasize their eyes. Additionally important for men: compared to mascara, tinted eyelashes and eyebrows always look more natural! Open your male customer's eyes!

The colour that squeezes out of the tube is not the end colour. So be sure you know your colours before tinting a client. Most tint suppliers can either sell you a company's tint chart or organize one to be sent to you.

THE IMPORTANCE OF A SALON BELL.

When I place eyelash tint on a client or for any other treatment where they need to lay there I place a small bell in their hand and place that hand on their stomach. I explain that if they have any issues they should ring the bell to draw my attention. Ask them not to touch their eyes and not to open their eyes nor try to get up.

Tell them to ring that bell and someone will be here to assist you in a flash.

Yes! all of us were told in beauty school not to leave the client unattended. But who in this day and age can afford to sit by a clients side for twenty minutes or more. I have three timers set.

The first one is set to check client in five minutes. A lot can happen in five minutes. Some clients get an itch, scratch their eyes, and put tint on another part on their face or body.

The second timer is set to check on her in ten minutes so that one is set for fifteen minutes. Then I ask if she would like to give the tint some more time. If her response is "yes" I set the timer for another ten minutes.

On the other hand, if the client is having Reflexology or some other treatment where I am in the room I set the first timer for twelve minutes and the second timer for another twenty minutes.

The longer her tint is on the longer it will last. Even if I am staying in the room, I give her/him the bell to hold. You may be called to check on another client, or called away for some other reason. Develop good foolproof plans and you will be less inclined to make mistakes or forget about a client.

Never say "Never" we all at some point in our working life make unbelievable mistakes no matter how astute we are.

Another point to consider is what if someone in your family is suddenly rushed to hospital and you need to leave the salon immediately.

Your junior or work colleagues will know exactly where you are up to with the client because you have at least two timers in the treatment room. The client has a bell and will ring it if she realizes she has been forgotten, or she is uncomfortable or if the tint is oozing into her eyes.

The other point is if the client is in the beauty slant position during the treatment once the treatment is on she may need to have her pillows readjusted for better comfort.

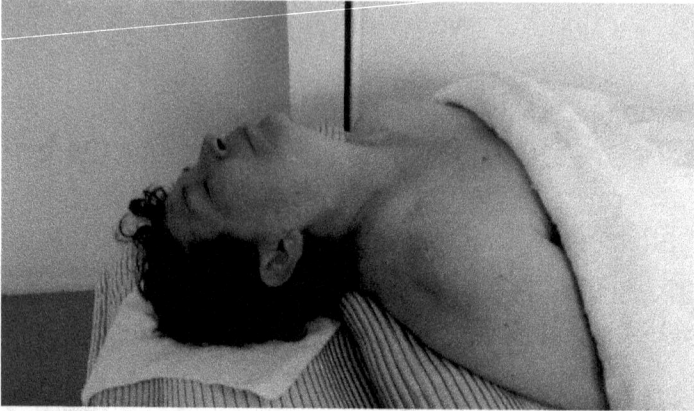

The beauty slant position is a safe position for the client but can be uncomfortable if not set up correctly.

- Place a small pillow under their knees
- Another small pillow in the small arch in their back.
- A large pillow under their shoulders and head.
- Then another pillow on top of that pillow which you place under their shoulders . This pillow allows the head to tilt back.

PATCH TEST HOW TO

After the client has been consulted and filled in his/her forms:

- Place a dark towel around her neck and secure it with a clip.
- Clip the hair behind both ears up.
- Take a photo of the area to be tinted
- Clean a small patch of skin behind the ears.
- Mix a tiny amount of eyelash and eyebrow tint as per mixing instructions. Each dye/tint must be mixed in a separate bowl.
- Apply a tiny dot of tint behind the ears
- Place the eyebrow tint behind one ear and the eyelash tint behind the other ear.
- Set your timer for ten minutes.
- Give the client the bell so she can ring it for help if it starts to burn her skin.
- Give the client a book or a cup of tea/coffee/water.
- Remove the tint with lukewarm water.
- Pat dry.
- Take the after treatment shot. It is important that the client holds her client card near the photo. This way there can never be a question as to which client the photo belongs to.

- Set up a time for the client to return the next day.
- If there was no reaction then the client can have the treatments. If there was a reaction, then you need to address the situation and place a large red warning sign on the clients history card.

ADDRESSING ADVERSE PATCH TEST.

RASH:-

If the clients has a rash, you need to apply an antiseptic lotion, oil or cream. These should be available for the client to purchase from you.

BLISTER:-

If the client has a blistering place an ice pack in paper towel. Have the client lay in a position where the ice pack will press on the skin without the need of holding it there for 10 minutes.

Pat dry very gently. Dab on an antiseptic oil.

Advise the client she needs to apply the ice pack three times a day. Drink two litres of water during the day. Apply the antiseptic cream twice a day. Only allow lukewarm or preferably cold water to touch that area while bathing.

ANTIHISTAMINE.

The client should be advised, to take an antihistamine. Do not recommend one to her. She will need to speak with the Chemist at her local pharmacy/drug store to enquire as to which brand would best suit her. They will question her about other medications she might be taking. They might even suggest she do to her Doctor.

EYE MAKE-UP REMOVER INFO

Before each eyelash and eyebrow tinting, the hair should be treated with the non-oily Refectocil Eye Make-Up Remover. That is particularly important because the hairs of the client must be oil free and clean of any make-up residue in preparation for tinting. Only then the best possible and long-lasting tinting result can be achieved. naturally here we are referring to their natural body oils. In some cases and almost all hot wax types of wax require an oil be applied before applying the wax.

However, I love Jojoba oil with a few drop of Chamomile essential oil added. It will never harm delicate eye tissue and in fact, will heal all eye conditions and improve skin texture. After the oil treatment, I then use a warm wet cloth and then a mild toner.

You can purchase this mix from all Essential oil companies. The bottle will usually say Chamomile and then in the fine print they add

"3% Jojoba Oil."

Now do they mean 3% of the bottle is Jojoba? No they mean 3% is Chamomile, and the rest of the bottle is Jojoba oil. What you need to purchase is:

CHAMOMILE ROMAN or CHAMOMILE GERMAN PURE ESSENTIAL OIL 6% with Jojoba Oil in a 10ml bottle. It comes with an eyedropper for ease of use. You are better advised to buy 10 ml of pure Chamomile plus an empty brown bottle with an eyedropper as the lid of the bottle.

In the empty bottle put 7 ml of Olive or Jojoba and 3 ml of the pure Chamomile oil.

You place two drops on each eyelid and gently massage that in.

All reputable Essential oil companies offer safety data sheets. When you click on the oil on their website, they have another option for more info. There message usually looks like this.

"For any enquiries in regards to MSDS (Material Safety Data Sheets) or COFA (Certificate of Analysis) documents please email your account manager or email us at nda@newdirections.com.au"

Am I advertising New Directions? NO. but I do buy my oils from them and have done so for many years.

LONG LASH GEL

Coloured hair must be regularly treated with a conditioner. Not only coloured hair, needs special care, but also tinted lashes and brows. Inform your clients of the importance for regular care, after brow and lash tinting. Some companies recommend to them the specifically developed care gel enriched with Vitamin E and D-Panthenol.

Coconut oil is an amazing lash ointment. I like to add one drop of Chamomile essential oil to one teaspoon of coconut oil and apply to my eye area each night.

BLEACHING PASTE.

Refectocil bleaching paste No.0 blonde lightens eyebrows up to 3 levels:

- To match too prominent or dark eyebrows with dyed blonde hair

- To achieve the desired natural colour (4N to 9N) as basis before tinting with Refectocil No. 4 chestnut and No. 4.1 red

BLEACHING EYEBROWS

Bleaching to match too prominent or dark eyebrows with dyed blonde hair.

Clients with dyed blonde hair, whose natural hair colour is black or brown, will be surprised! In the past "false blondes" could easily be exposed because of their too prominent or dark eyebrows. This belongs to the past as eyebrows can now be lightened by up to 3 levels with Refectocil Bleaching paste for eyebrows No. 0 blonde and as a result will match perfectly with the shade of bleached/dyed blonde hair. Never ever use hair bleach.

BLEACHING BEFORE TINTING WITH REDS

Bleaching before tinting with Refectocil No. 4 chestnut and No. 4.1 red

By using Refectocil No. 0 blonde to bleach eyebrows before tinting with No. 4 chestnut and No. 4.1 red you can achieve a variety of red and auburn colours, no matter what your client's natural hair colour is.

Refectocil No. 4 chestnut and No. 4.1 red can be used without prior bleaching for natural colours from 4N to 9N. For natural colours 1N to 3N use Refectocil No.0 blonde before tinting with No.4 chestnut or No. 4.1 red in order to achieve 4N or lighter, as desired. Cleanse the eyebrows after the bleaching with the non-oily Refectocil Eye Make-Up Remover, because eyebrows must be free of oil and dry, so that with the following application of Refectocil tint an optimum tinting result can be obtained.

ASH BLONDE CLIENTS

How to get a suitable colour for Ash blonde clients that find the 3.1 Light Brown too red

Mix 3.1 Light Brown with 1.1 Graphite at a ratio of 1:1 to obtain a toned down, ashen hue.

MIXING OF TINT COLOURS

Fundamentally you can mix all Refectocil colours – with the exception of Refectocil No. 4 chestnut - with one another. However, we recommend this only to experienced users!

With the available Refectocil colours, a multiplicity of shades can be achieved and almost all clients wishes fulfilled. Please note; that Refectocil No. 4 chestnut under no circumstances should be mixed with other Refectocil colours! In addition, you should never mix Refectocil eyelash and eyebrow tints with other eyelash and eyebrow brands.

UNDERSTANDING COLOURS

During a hairdressers training period, they learn a great deal about colour. Should they become a colour specialist they have to attend extra courses and have that added to their License. These days they call it a Diploma in Colour and become a Colour Technician.

Unfortunately, the module on colour in Beauty Therapy is somewhat inadequate. Therefore, I have taken the liberty to refresh your memory on colour mixing and hope it is enough information for you to understand reflects of eyebrow and eyelash colours.

First we need to understand the Natural hair colour range. They are referred to as "N".

N1 is Black   N9 is Blonde

The lower the number the darker the colour.

Depth	Number	Shade
Lightest	10	*Lightest blonde*
	9	*Very light blonde*
	8	*Light blonde*
Mid Range	7	*Blonde*
	6	*Dark blonde*
	5	*Light brown*
	4	*Brown*
Darkest	3	*Dark brown*
	2	*Very dark brown*
	1	*Black*

Some clients always shoot red reflects and need "Ash tint" added to their tint. If they do not like the red highlights showing in their hair, when they stand in bright lights or the sun. Unfortunately, the size of this book prevents me from giving you a clear chart to have a look at. However, you can go onto any of the major hairdressing websites to view a colour chart.

http://media.wella.com/professional/m/pdf/WCC_Education_Book-English.pdf

With hair tints, we use a tint that has "A" attached to its colour number which means "Ash" and ash kills the red reflections.

Even when a client has completely white hair they can shoot red and gold reflects.

You would naturally think that bleach lightens hair colour no matter what colour the hair is.

That is not completely correct. When you apply bleach or a lightening tint to white or platinum blonde hair it becomes darker. The white or platinum blonde hair turns golden blonde. Then something more permanent starts to happen. Once you put any kind of peroxide on their skin/scalp .

The chart below indicates bleaching dark hair to lighter shades. Bear in mind though that the skin structure and the eyebrow hairs react differently to the hair on our head. The strength of the peroxide/developer needs to be much lower for the eyebrows.

Warning. If this is the first time a client has come to you, you need to do a pack test before you bleach. If they say they have had it done before with no problems you can skip the patch test but you need to have then sign, a disclaimer form and an honesty statement *more on that later.*

This is what happened to this young dancer.

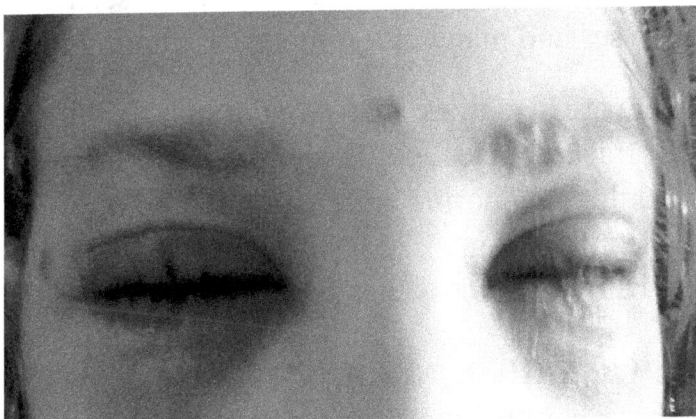

The teenager was also left partially blind. Her father said: 'When it all went wrong, I was shocked that they didn't even apologize.

Follow us: @MailOnline on Twitter | DailyMail on Facebook

Makeup artists do not have a diploma in Beauty. It only takes a few hours to get a Certificate to apply eyelash and brow tints. I do hope that International Standard changes before I go to meet my maker.'

In hindsight, I say they did **not** do a patch test on Masha Kuznetsov, a promising young dancer, now scared for life.

It is because of cases like these that I write these training manuals. There are too many people thinking," I can do that myself", and far too many trades that cross over and miss that most important parts of training. Skin anatomy, skin science, scalp analyses and many other important training modules.

There are also those that skip through their training in fast track courses and those that think the important modules are boring and know that if they fail the subject they don't like it does not matter as they will get better marks in other subject to gain a pass.

Always do a patch test. Never allow children to have hair, eyebrow, and eyelash tints. Never do them on people with sensitive skin.

If you are a home user reading this book so you can create your own beautiful eyebrows and lashes please do a patch test first.

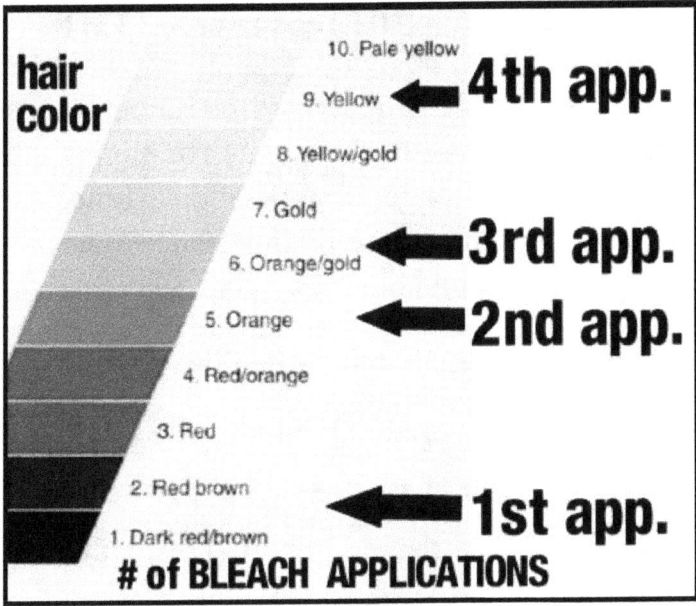

CORRECT APPLICATION TIME.

The application time is different from client to client; it depends on the hair of the client. The tinting effect increases with longer application time. The application time in general is up to ten minutes, with Refectocil browns and blacks.

No. 4 chestnut, No. 4.1 red.

No.0. blonde leave up to 20 minutes to process.

If you do not have very much experience with tinting, remove the tinting paste after 10-12 minutes from one eyebrow and check the result and/or show the client. If the tinting result is not intensive enough yet, apply the tinting paste again and leave longer.

However, I have added my personal notes elsewhere in this book. I need at least forty-five minutes for my tint as I have fine hair and lashes.

EYEBROW TINT APPLICATION

After a Successful patch test:-

Take a photo of the clients face.

If the client come, into the salon with makeup and mascara applied, you will need to remove it. The client should have been asked to come in with a clean face at the time of her making an appointment. If the client chose to wear makeup she needs to be advised you will need to do a mini facial and advised of the cost.

I use a 1cm or ¾ inch of tint with 6 drops of developer/Oxidant. The larger bottle in the next photo is the one I like.

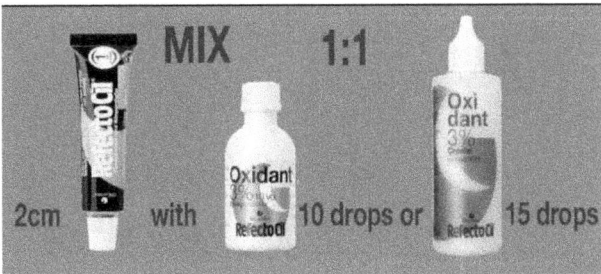

MIX 1:1
2cm with Oxidant 10 drops or 15 drops

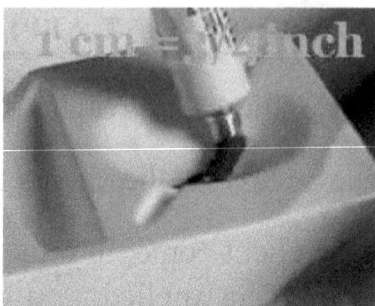

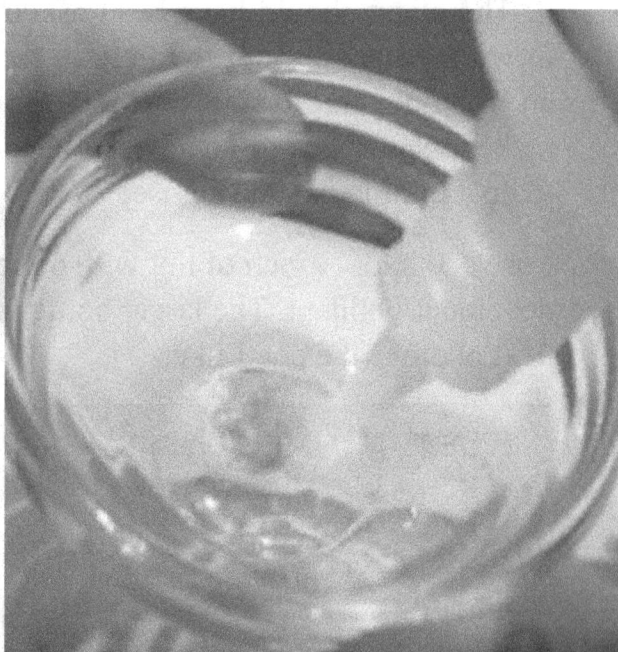

Mix well with a small stiff lipstick brush. The colour will darken as you mix the product together. Mix well to a smooth thick paste.

1. Once you and the client have decided on a colour and you have filled in the form.

2. Take a photo of her eyebrows.

3. Place a headband on her head.

4. Place a black towel over her neck and chest.

5. Place paper towel over the pillow.

6. Place a pillow under her shoulders so her head titles back into the beauty slant position.

7. Wash your hands, dry and put on gloves. Never put the gloves on until you begin her treatment.

8. Clean her brows twice.

9. Decide on the shape and pencil them in with a sterilized pencil.

10. Now apply an oil to the outsides of the eyebrow shape.

11. Place about one-quarter of an inch or half a centimetre of the tint in your glass dish with a few drops of peroxide/developer, mix to a thick paste.

12. Apply the tint to the eyebrow hair from the outer edge towards the nose then apply in the opposite direction. Only apply to the shape of the brow.

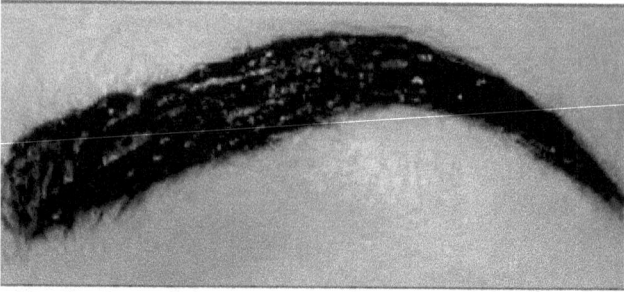

13.

14. I like to ask the client to sit on their hands. This prevents them from touching the brow while waiting ten to twenty minutes for it to process.

15. Remove the tint with a wet cotton pad be sure to fold the pad so you do not put tint on their skin as you remove it from their brows.

16. Repeat the process until the brow is soft and clean.

17. Then apply a skin toner.

18. Wet a cotton pad, apply toner to the pad and in a press and lift motion tone the eyebrows

19. Next apply Chamomile oil. Chamomile oil is best purchased mixed with Jojoba oil.

~ * ~

EYEBROW EXTENSIONS.

In this book, I will give some brief notes on eyebrow extensions. However, I intend to add these to my eyelash extension book because that is where I think eyebrow extensions is best placed.

Glues and the skins reactions to glue is covered in my Book

Eyelash Extensions Grafted Lashes Training Manual

The new book to be released late 2016 Is probably going to be called " Eyelash and Eyebrow Extensions."

In brief it is very easy to add hairs to the eyebrows.

They last for five to twenty days.

You use the same type and amount of glue as you do for eyelash extensions.

Before

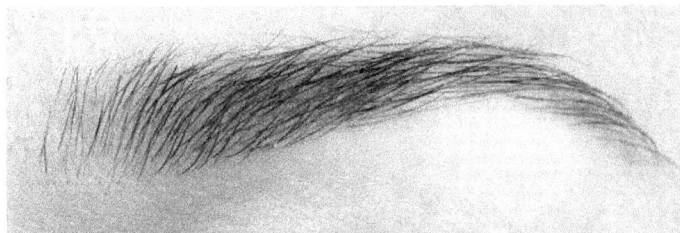

After Waxing and Adding Hair

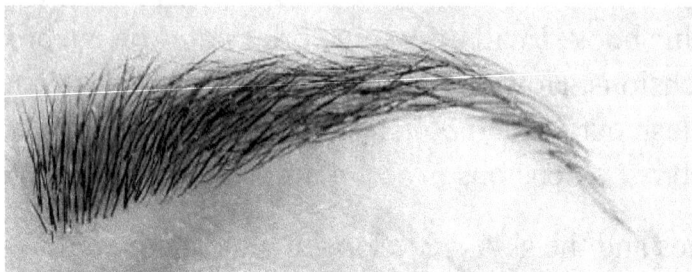

Attach each new hair to an existing hair.

You should be well trained in eyelash extensions before you train in eyebrow extensions.

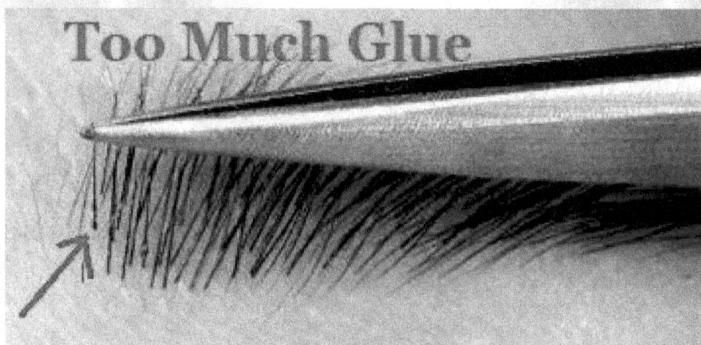

Too Much Glue

When you pick up the extension hair and dip it in the glue wipe the tip of the extension on foil or the side of the bowl, before you attach it to the eyebrow hair. There should not be a knob of glue

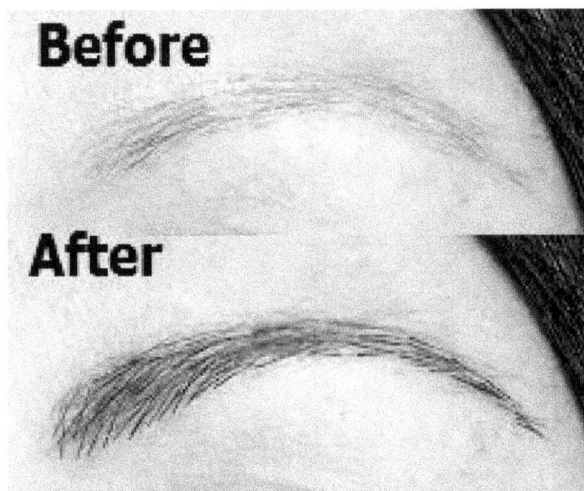

where the extension meets the eyebrow hair.

From a distance, the above photo would look OK but up close and personal, this would look terrible. The hair thickness was too thick. Only buy your eyebrow hair from suppliers that have a good reputation. However, when you look at the bald patches in the before photo this client was happy with the results. Nevertheless, girls with practice you can do better than this.

Practice on raw pig skin first. Buy some false eyebrows sick on the pigskin and practice.

Keeping the skin under the brow tinted weekly is very important, as you will gauge in the next

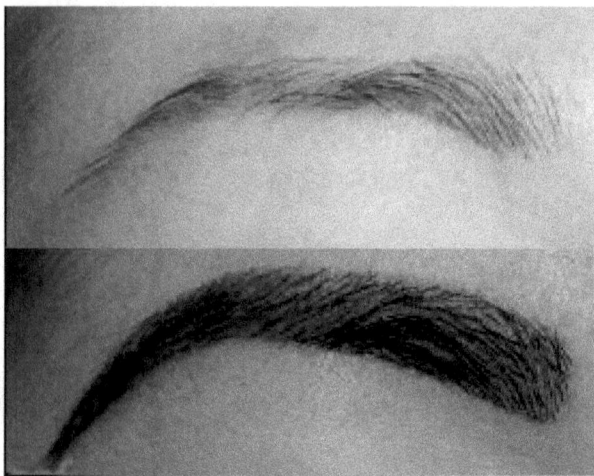

photo.

~ * ~

EYEBOW DIP

Eyebrow dip is a cream product that comes in a few shades. I advocate using two colours for a more natural appearance. I recommend these videos on YouTube

https://www.youtube.com/watch?v=elZ9i-PULdQ

Try to buy a trio pack with two shades of brown and a concealer, and an eyebrow contour brush.

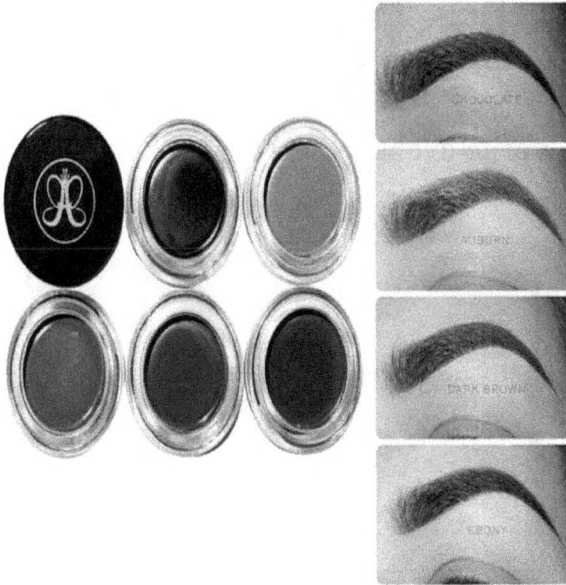

You can get these products on eBay. Eyebrow mascara is also a very helpful product for those of you that have great eyebrows and simply just need more depth to your eyebrows.

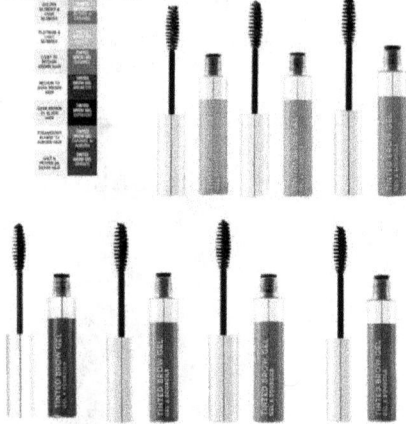

My Favorite eyebrow powder brush.

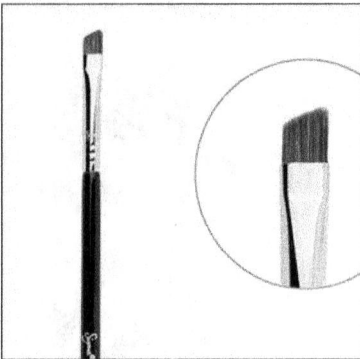

A WORD FROM THE AUTHOR

Hello all,

Many, many, moons ago when I began waxing, in those days (1950's to 1970's) we made our own wax. There were no other options as non of the suppliers sold wax.

We also saved the wax, boiled it and put through a sieve to remove everyone's hair. Then we reheated the wax and reused it. In some parts of the world to this very day they still do it that way. However eyebrows were seldom waxed. The client either had their eyebrows:-

- Plucked every week

- Removed by an epilator

- Removed with fine sandpaper.

- Shaved

- Removed by string wrapped around each hair. Called "THREADING"

In today world lots of people still use these old methods in various forms. In fact some people need to employ these older methods for various reasons. They might be allergic to wax or its by-products.

They may have very dry skin and find sandpapering works best to give the skin around the eyebrows a softer look. The older methods may suit their lifestyle better. Maybe some live in remote areas where they do not have access to beauty products nor a beauty therapist.

After owning and running Hairdressing and Beauty Salons for over 50 years I have seen many changes in the industry. Some great and some not so great.

With each of my training manuals, my hope is to assist the future generations to improve their skills. While at technical college or a beauty school sometimes you are so consumed, with all that you need to learn, you miss the finer points. No one can ever remember every single thing, they are taught. These manuals are to assist those of you that:

Want to be the best in the business and improve your skills.

Want to return to the industry after a break.

Want to do your own beauty treatments at home.

Either way, the most important facts to becoming an expert are to:-

- Read and reread and reread everything on each application.

- Practice and practice and re-practice until you have it down pat and feel very confident.

- Look at photos of people and study their face. Are their eyebrows the right shape and colour for their face and complexion?

- Draw eyebrows onto pork skin and practice waxing

- Keep practising on some kind of practice sheet or animal skin until you are amazingly confident.

- Take before and after photos of your own eyebrows and the eyebrows of everyone, you know.

Produced and written by Robyna Smith-Keys

Email beautyschoolbooks@gmail.com

Beauty School Books Learning Academe

Beauty School Books is an online beauty school. Servicing students with their elective studies, for the hairdressing and beauty industry. We assist people returning to work to reinforce their skills. As well, we assist those that could not afford to enrol in the elective studies while at college. Nothing can match going to college to learn and feed knowledge off other students. However, when that is not an option we are here to help.

Email beautyschoolbooks@gmail.com
http://www.beautyschoolbooks.com
The website offers:-
Beauty tips

Beauty School Training Manuals

Body Piercing

Hairstyles

Dreadlocks

Fashion Tips And More

ASSOCIATIONS TO JOIN

ASSOCIATION OF PROFESSIONAL AUSTRALIA AESTHETICIANS.

Telephone 07 5575 9364 Email

info@apaa.com.au | www.apaa.com.au

P.O BOX 96 ROBINA QLD 4226

> I also am a member of APAA they have been in business now for 53 years so they are doing something right. Their website is loaded with adverts and they are the ones that the Government

asked to write the Australian Standards. In 1992 and then they commissioned me and many other therapists to assist with the setting up of the Australian standards.

Then again in 2007 - 2014 Australia was invited to write the International Standards. The writing of the international Standard was organized by
Services Industries Skills Council
Level 10, 171 Clarence St
Sydney NSW 2001
Phone: +61 2 8243 1210   Fax: +61 2 8243 1299
www.serviceskills.com.au e-mail:
info@serviceskills.com.au

I do hope you found this book helpful and welcome your feedback. Constructive criticism is how we grow and improve.

OTHER BOOKS BY
ROBYNA SMITH-KEYS

HEALING AND TRAINING MANUALS

Foolproof Aromatherapy

Essential oils can heal, sooth and energize. Learn how to mix, when not to use and all the benefits for hundreds of ailments listed in alphabetical order. User-friendly.

The Antique Healer

This is a much large Aromatherapy book with photos and more healings. Also, contains wise old women's remedies.

I Was Not Ready To Lose My Mother

My mother had a few weeks to live. Her cancer was very aggressive. I set her up on a healing program of juices, essential oils and herbs. This was all working until she stopped the program. It also has a lovely storey about her life. Married at age 16 until her Passover at 83 years of age.

Organic Cancer Cure

This cure helped my mother it might help you.

HOW TO TRAINING MANUALS.

Body Piercing Basics

All the main points on body piercing.

Anatomy For Body Piercers

All body piercers should understand the body and how it works. This is a wonderful tool for any body piercer.

Eyelash Extensions Grafted Lashes Training Manual

Step by step instructions with video tutorials.

Eyebrows Shaping And Tinting To Suit Face Shapes

Step by step instructions with video tutorials on eyebrow shaping, eyelash and brow tinting.

Cosmetic Tattoo Permanent Makeup Micro-pigmentation

A training manual with step by step instruction. Students have said, you could actually teach yourself the trade as this book is so well written.

An Angel For Cosmetic tattooist

A Permanent Makeup Bible. The helping hand for a cosmetic tattooist. It has every this the training manual has except the exams. You will not need to gather information from anywhere else.

HAIR EXTENSIONS TRAINING MANUAL

Learn to create hair wefts, weaves, braids, wax in, and clip in Hair Extensions. There are videos to watch in the eBook.

SUPERNATURAL & SELF HELP BOOKS:-

BA HA HA HAPPY!

A great way to start a journey into feeling marvelously alive.

POSITIVE SPIRITUAL AFFIRMATIONS

Loaded with helpful veres mediation and healings of the mind.

Colours That Heal.

Every colour has an effect on your life learn what they are and do.

SPELL FOLKLORE

A great book on how to do some positive affirmations also called spells.

TAROT SCROLLS 0-22

Ask a question open a page and an inspiring answer will be there for you to read.

CHILDREN'S BOOKS:-

ROMEO AND JULIETTE KEEP MARK ANTONY

A wonderful storey about a puppy born on a boat. His white cute and fluffy. A true storey with a dash of magic added.

MARK ANTONY MARRIES LIZY AND HAS PUPPIES

Loaded with photos of all the dogs and the new born puppies. A true story with a dash of fantasy added.

###

Gather friend to practice on and enjoy your new journey.

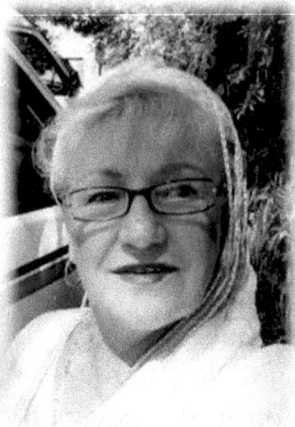

With Love From

Robyna XOX